MILK ...
to drink,
or not to drink ??

MILK ...
To drink,
or not to drink ??

Brent Bateman
Bsc, Msc Human Nutrition

Part Four of the series:
The Nutrition Factor:
A Bold New Perspective

September, 2010

ACKNOWLEDGEMENTS

Acknowledge is respectfully given to the vast input over the course of human history .... to all those who have contributed to the knowledge and understanding of human nutrition .... and especially to the scientists, health care professionals, and individuals who have strived for increased knowledge and enhanced understanding in more recent times.

DEDICATION

This book is dedicated first to the quest for improvement of mankind's condition through greater knowledge and better understanding of human nutrition.

Secondly, this series is addressed and dedicated to the general public, who has the right to insist on correct nutritional information and the right to require that the professional health care community, the food industry, and government, act responsibly, with integrity and transparency, to insure that the public is properly informed and served.

FOREWORD

Is there a crack in our food pyramid ??

The author tells us "yes, there is a crack in our food pyramind" ... in fact, not only one, but there are several.

Explaining these 'cracks' is one way to introduce the author's series: *The Nutrition Factor: A Bold New Perspective.* In Part One of the series the author challenges the paradigm statement that "we can obtain all our necessary nutrients by consuming a variety of basic foods and maintaining a balanced diet". Part Two analyzes our food supply in a historical perspective and explains its limitations and inadequacies. The author then leads from these two beginning premises to present a 'bold new perspective', critically reviewing much of the 'conventional wisdom' in nutrition and medicine. This book is written ahead of the first three because of the importance and urgency of the subject matter and message. But it is perhaps appropriate, because the case of cow's milk is an excellent example of a food that is relatively new in a historical sense, but in the last one hundred and fifty years has been promoted as "nature's most perfect food", and is currently highly regarded as an important food choice for modern humans ...yet it is also the source of much controversy. It is a good starting point for the series.

Very recent scientific investigation has revealed that cow's milk can be separated into two main categories, based on its chemical composition ... designated as A1 and A2 ... and that A1 milk contains a highly disruptive molecule, BCM-7, which may trigger biological pathways that are directly linked to diabetes, heart disease, schizophrenia, autism, and even sudden-death-syndrome.

A note on the author's style of writing

The author has been long dismayed by the sorts of writing presented by various authors on the subject of nutrition.

His discomfort has been the most extreme when reading books or articles by self-proclaimed nutrition experts, usually with an MD attached to their surname, that attempt to convince us that this one magic substance is an absolute cure for multiple illnesses ... or that he or she is the one and only valid source of correct nutrition information. It seems that most of us harbor a propensity to favor this kind of approach, and these authors take advantage of that weakness. This type of thinking is especially prevalent among proponents of 'health foods' and alternative solutions. The goal of these writers is usually to make a lot of money.

On the other side of the spectrum, nutrition scientists and health care professionals fail to write in language and terminology that is understood by the general public ... if indeed they address their writing to the public at all. Scientists and academics notoriously write to themselves, or among themselves, with little attention to trying to inform the public.

One often hears the complaint: "What is correct ... is this good to eat ... or not ?" or "Who do I believe ?" In almost all writing addressed to the public there is the additional annoyance of the authors not identifying their references, sources, or support for their conclusions, plus embracing a strong bias ... there is little in the way of an attempt to 'give both sides of the story' and either let the reader make their own decisions, or lead them to more substantiated conclusions.

He has therefore tried something different. First, he has attempted to remain objective, and not fall sway to the urge to draw strong conclusions or to sensationalize, or to resort to 'belief'. He has, secondly, included references and supporting literature in the text, with comments. Thirdly, he has attempted to present the different points of view and opposing conclusions presented by the multitude of literary sources and their authors, with the goal of 'showing the different sides of the story'. His own conclusions are offered tentatively, leaving room for the reader to draw their own conclusions, and honoring the long-learned lesson that 'no conclusions are valid until all the evidence is in' which almost never happens ... such is the nature of scientific investigation.

A fresh perspective

This book approaches the question of whether or not we should drink cow's milk from a fresh perspective ... a fresh perspective made possible by two recent, separate events. First, the broad scope of available data providing the nutrient content of cow's milk is relatively new ... the current USDA data base for food composition, SR 22, 2009, was expanded to include 13 of the 14 essential vitamins, and 10 of the 20 to 22 minerals known to be essential to humans ... this is an update from the 2005 SR 18, which only supplied information for 9 vitamins and 9 minerals. Our knowledge about milk has also benefited from an array of recent studies and research efforts which have greatly expanded our current understanding.

Secondly, this approach attempts to find a 'middle path' between the extreme advocacies of 'milk is the perfect food' and the opposite: 'milk is totally bad for us'. The point of view that milk is nature's most perfect food grew out of a century and a half of the rise of milk-drinking to become a traditional and popular American habit ... the opposing anti-milk point of view is more recent, and is founded in a reaction to such things as the use of 'recombinant bovine growth hormone' (rBGH), and the growth of the vegetarian and animal rights cults. In this respect the author attempts to follow what Melanie DuPuis describes in her wonderful book *Nature's Perfect Food* as the 'imperfect story'.

TABLE OF CONTENTS

CHAPTER ONE

INTRODUCTION AND OVERVIEW

Is there a crack in our food pyramid ??

Although the USDA and the folks who put together our national food guidelines are improving their format to allow for alternatives to milk and dairy products as part of their recommendations, the old thinking still prevails.

So ... should Americans consume 2, 3, or even 4 servings of milk and milk products each day? Even though some of us are vegans, and refuse to touch the stuff. Or are animal rights sympathizers and don't purchase dairy products because they come from animals. Almost one hundred percent of adult Native Americans cannot digest milk products due to genetic lactose intolerance, as are 90% Asian-Americans, 75% African-Americans, 69% Jewish-Americans, 53% American Hispanics, and 15% Caucasian-Americans. Does the wide dark-blue band in the food pyramid apply to these people as well? Or, many Americans do not want to consume milk that is from cows treated with recombinant bovine growth hormone (rBGH), excessive anti-biotics, and other such things ... and current labeling laws do not *require* that milk from treated cows be labeled as such, and in some states it is actually against the law to label milk as coming from rBGH-free cows. Does the food pyramid guidelines apply to these concerned folks as well? How about new evidence that maybe all that calcium that we get from dairy products really doesn't give us healthy bones? And now there are rumors that the consumption of cow's milk is linked to several disease conditions in human, including diabetes, heart disease, neurological dysfunction, and even a couple of cancers.

Yes, maybe there is a crack in our food pyramid !!

So the questions beg being asked: Is milk truly "natures most perfect food? Does it really contain high quantities of many essential vitamins and minerals? So, what about calcium and protein? And what about its fat content? Is milk fat harmful for us? How about omega 3, and iron, and vitamin C? What about the bioavailability of the nutrients? Should we be feeding cow's milk to babies and infants? Does drinking milk help to lower the risk of some chronic diseases? What about claimed links with allergies, inflammation, and even breast cancer? What about 'lactose

1

intolerance', or the other side of the same coin, 'lactase deficiency'? Now we hear about the substance called BCM-7 … is this really bad for us? How credible is the evidence? What can be done about it … if it truly *is* so harmful? If nothing is being done, why? And who is responsible?

Purpose

The purpose of this in-depth review is to (a) inform you, the reader and the public, of the many pros and cons of this important issue, (b) to present new scientific data which identifies a health-damaging molecule in type A1 cow's milk and the biological mechanism which links this substance to the onset of diabetes and other chronic disease conditions, and (c) to prompt a call for action to mediate the dangers and hold accountable those who knowingly have deceived the public.

My intent is *not* to finally lay this vast controversy to rest … this cannot be done, because there is still so much that we do not know. It is hoped, however, that this treatise will help to stimulate thought and discussion, more research, and a call to action.

Rationale

There has been a great deal written and debated over the years regarding the question about whether cow's milk is a suitable food for human consumption. However, much of the argument has been strongly biased. This bias has originated from a variety of sources. High consumption of milk, as one example, is strongly based on religious beliefs in some cultures. Or, milk has been so highly exonerated in some countries due to its perceived health benefits that to question its merits is deemed folly and mischievous. Or, an intensely profit-orientated and politically powerful dairy industry has bombarded the public for several life-times with pro-milk advertising, outright propaganda, and directed research. There has been a dismal lack of objective and critical inquiry, and little discussion that has included all the points of view. The author suggests that the strength of the pro-milk bias in Western cultures is so overwhelming that this bias has become embedded in the 'conventional wisdom' of nutrition and dietetics, and is a part of the prevailing paradigm of western medicine and health care as a whole.

In contrast, there has emerged a more recent 'anti-milk movement' nurtured by events such as the growth of the vegetarian cult, and the popularity of the animal rights movement, a reaction to artificial and big-business interventions such as the use of 'recombinant bovine growth hormone' (rBGH), the consensus that human breast milk is far superior for feeding our babies, and increasing evidence of links with a number of disease conditions in humans.

Attempting to resolve this complex dilemma, then, becomes the rationale for this treatise, which seeks a more rational and objective 'midlle-road' perspective.

Presentation

I have attempted something different in the writing of this book. First, I try to be as objective as I can, presenting each point of view and argument as fairly as possible. Secondly, I have included important references and comments in the text, with a reference summary at the ends of each chapter ... with the hope that this will allow the reader to follow the supporting evidence more closely and with a clearer understanding. Finally, I try to present the opposing studies and evidence separately, providing room for the reader to view the opposing evidence and formulate his own conclusions.

At the end of Chapter Two, the "Good" and Chapter Three, the "Bad", I have listed the references used in the text, and then I have also included a separate section that presents additional references for each of the sub-headings, with conclusions and comments. The intent is to offer the reader the chance to survey a sampling of the available literature and research. If the reader cares to take the time, and is of course interested, these references can allow for a broader perspective of the pros and cons, and provide a better base to make an individual appraisal.

How we came to have the cow and cow' milk

All domestic cattle, and the *cow*, are descended from the ancient primordial ox, or the *auroch*, with the scientific name *Bos primigenius* (first cow). All of the humpless cattle in the Western world are of the more recent sub-species *Bos Taurus*, and the humped cattle coming from the Indian sub-continent are from the *bos indicus*. The now-extinct auroch was a truly massive beast, nearly twice the size of the largest modern cow, and with fierceness equal to that of the lion or bear. Julius Caesar, speaking of rare encounters with the few aurochs remaining in the wild during his era, judged that they were about the size of small elephants, and to be able to kill one immortalized a hunter. (A Cow's Life, 2004)

So domestication must surely have been a long and challenging process, with the auroch first being hunted and then held in captivity for their meat, hides, and bones, and were slowly bred over many generations for softer temperaments and smaller size. Domestication to the degree to allow humans to remove milk from their udders did not occur until about 7,000 years ago, and the first cows produced less than one quart of milk per day. The average daily production for all dairy cows in the U.S. in 2005 was 26.8 quarts (24.1 liters). The art of milking cows has come a long way.

An introduction to cow's milk

Milk is the opague white liquid produced by the mammary glands of mammals, and universally provides the primary source for young mammals before they are able to digest other types of food. The milk of each species is therefore specific for that species. In other words, the make-up of the milk of each animal is different, and reflects the special needs of that species. Humans are the only animal species that consumes the milk of other animals, and continue to do so past the infant weaning stage, and into adulthood. As an example, calves … the infant young of the cow … suckle their mother's mammary gland only to the age of approximately 3 months, when their weaning period ends. Young calves, once having reached the end of their weaning period, typically refuse the milk of their mothers and seek other foods. It is also noteworthy that the first milk for the newborn calf, 'colostrum', is very different from the milk produced later … it is heavy with extra nutrients and hormones designed to give the newborn its needed boost.

During our recent history, we humans have consumed the milk of many different animals, depending largely on which animals were available in each geographic area. These include the water buffalo, camel, horse, reindeer, donkey, and yak, plus the goat and sheep. In Russia and Sweden, small moose dairies still exist. More recently, we have found that the cross-breed of the cow and the bison also produce large quantities of milk.

The ability to capture the milk from domesticated animal udders was unquestionably a major event in the evolution of human populations and culture. There is a great deal written on this subject, and I will come back to it in the next chapter, but at this point it is important to note that recent studies in anthropology and genetics have shown that the ability to successfully consume the milk of other animals enabled human populations to survive and multiply much more effectively. Dr. Sarah Tishkoff and her team from the University of Maryland have calculated that the ability to use milk as a source of food nutrition may have contributed to population growth as much as ten times, compared with populations which did not consume animal milk. (Wade, 2006

There are two grades of milk commonly produced in the United States. Grade A is used for direct consumption and sold in retail outlets; Grade B is used for indirect consumption via processing and the formation of secondary products such as cheeses. Dairy farms are divided according to whether they produce Grade A or Grade B milk. The following are the general regulatory guidelines:

❖ Grade A farms are inspected every 6 months, Grade B farms every 2 years.

❖ Both types of farms are required to have two cleaning vats in the milkhouse for washing and rinsing of equipment, and must also have an additional separate sink and faucet for hand washing.

❖ Grade A milk is stored in a bulk tank cooled to 45 degrees Fahrenheit within 3 hours of milking. The maximum allowed temporary rise in temperature due to adding milk to the tank is to 50 degrees.

❖ Grade B milk is usually stored in milk cans, and must be cooled to 50 degrees Fahrenheit within 2 hours of milking, and milk from previous milkings cannot be mixed.

❖ The somatic cell count (SCC) of Grade A or B milk must not exceed 750,000 cells per mL.

❖ The bacterial plate or 'loop count' of Grade A milk may not exceed 100,000 per mL, and Grade B milk must not exceed 300,000 per mL.

❖ A bacterial plate count test is required at least once a month. If the bacterial count exceeds the stipulated limit in 3 out of 5 tests, the license to sell milk is suspended ... and will be immediately revoked if the bacterial count should ever exceed 750,000 per mL.

The composition of milk

The following table lists the main constituents of cow's milk, with the range and average (mean) percent content by weight.

Constituent	Range (%)	Mean (%)
Water	85.5 – 89.5	87.0
Total solids	10.5 – 14.5	13.0
Fat	2.5 – 6.0	4.0
Proteins	2.9 – 5.0	3.4
Lactose	3.6 – 5.5	4.8
Minerals	0.6 – 0.9	0.8

Milk is basically a water-based fluid with 'globules' of butterfat, and 'micelles' (small groups of molecules) of protein ... both of which combine to form an 'emulsion', or 'colloid'. The complex sugar, lactose, is soluble with the water portion, forming a molecular solution.

Milk fats

Whole milk contains three types of fats: saturated fat (approximately 65% of the total fat), monounsaturated (about 29%), polyunsaturated (3.6%), and cholesterol (0.5%).

Milk carbohydrates (sugars), lactose

Lactose is a disaccharide sugar, made up of equal portions of the simple sugars glucose and galactose. In order for lactose to pass through the small intestine wall membranes it must first be cleaved into glucose and galactose, requiring the enzyme *lactase*. Lactose is the major carbohydrate in almost all animal milks, and most animal infants produce the enzyme lactase during their weaning period, enabling them to digest the milk lactose. However, the production of this enzyme normally declines sharply after the weaning period ... for all animals, including humans. Some human populations, or individuals, have adapted or have benefited from a genetic alteration which enables them to produce lactase after their infant weaning period, even into adulthood. *Not* producing the enzyme lactase after infancy is the *norm*. Most Asian, African, and Native American populations (including central and South America) are lactase deficient after infancy.

Calcium

Cow's milk is a particularly rich source of several minerals, most notably calcium ... plus phosphorous, zinc, and selenium. For each of these minerals a daily intake of equivalent to 4 servings would provide between 25 and 100% of the RDA guideline amounts. It also contains lesser amounts of iron, magnesium, potassium, sodium, copper, and manganese, in amounts ranging from 6 to 18% of the RDA with 4 servings.

The efficiency of absorption or the *bioavailability* of the nutrients in milk is known to be particularly high compared with other food sources. This is especially true for the proteins in milk and the minerals, most noticeably calcium. The reasons are not fully understood, but the presence of lactose and phosphorous is thought to be a reason, plus the observance that milk remains in the stomach and small intestines for a longer time than do most other food substances, thereby allowing absorption to take place more completely.

Protein

The importance of protein in nutrition cannot be understated. In fact, the word 'protein' is derived from the Greek, *proteos,* meaning 'primary', or 'taking place first'.

Proteins in foods become available for use by our human physiologies after they have been broken down into the component amino acids, of which nine are *essential*, or *indispensible* (the ninth, histidine, is essential only for infants). By essential, we mean that if we have zero intake, death will be the eventual outcome. In recent years, however, this definition has been softened to include 'conditionally essential' and 'acquired indispensability'. If a given protein contains all of the nine essential amino acids, it is then considered to be *complete*, although one or more of the amino acids may be in relatively short supply, and therefore can influence the total ability to be utilized ... these are dubbed *limiting* amino acids.

A central concept in protein metabolism is the 'amino acid pool(s)', which contains amino acids of dietary origin plus those contributed by the breakdown of body tissues. These pools of amino acids then become available to various cells in the body, to then be utilized in a large number of roles. These roles include: (a) forming contractile proteins, including 'actin' and 'myosin', found in muscle; (b) constructing fibrous proteins such as collagen, elastin, and keratin; (c) creating molecules that act as *enzymes* ... catalysts to change the rate of biochemical reactions; (d) as derivatives to form hormones; (e) forming immunoproteins; and (f) assisting in the transport of proteins; (g) to act as a 'buffer' to ameliorate changes in pH (acidity or alkalinity) of the blood and other body tissues;

7

and (h) to conjugate with other nonprotein compounds to form such entities as 'glycoproteins' and 'lipoproteins'.

The major protein in milk is *casein*, which comprises 76 to 86% of the milk protein, and is divided into alpha-casein, beta casein, and gamma casein, with alpha casein being the major portion (60% of the total casein). Alpha casein is further separated into 'alpha-s-casein' and 'k-casein'. The remaining 14 to 24% of the protein portion in milk is a variety of proteins collectively called 'whey proteins', of which *lactoglobulin* is the most common (7-12% of the total whey proteins). 'Whey' is also the technical term used to describe the conglomerate typically left behind when the caseins coagulate into 'curds'. The whey proteins are typically more water-soluble than the casein proteins, and do not form large structures. They are therefore more easily absorbed by the body, and are considered an exceptionally rich source of amino acids, some of which are less available from other sources.

The 'good', the 'bad', and the 'ugly

It is with a touch of humor that I apply the analogy of the *good*, the *bad*, and the *ugly* … which may be considered inappropriate considering the serious implications of the matter at hand … and yet, it fits. Cow's milk has long been argued to be "good" … the "perfect food" in fact. Yet a host of counter-arguments and culturally based perspectives view the consumption of cow's milk by humans to be "bad". Now, new evidence supports the notion that cow's milk, at least the major variety that is currently being marketed, is nothing less than "ugly".

The Good

Milk *can* be an important source of many essential nutrients, especially calcium and protein. It is readily available in cultures that have historically consumed milk, and is relatively inexpensive. Several associations have been suggested with decreased risk of various chronic diseases, and with weight control. Complaints of lactose intolerance and links to allergies, inflammation, and breast cancer may be either exaggerated or based on wrong information.

The Bad

Milk was not a food choice for ancestral humans … domestication of the cow sufficient to extract milk from its udder did not take place until about 7,000 years ago, and drinking large quantities of liquid milk did not become popular until the middle of the 19th century, and particularly after the invention of pasteurization in the 1920s. Because of this, and other factors, one could argue that cow's milk is designed for the cow, not for humans. Vegan and animal rights proponents argue that our food choices should be derived from plants, not other animal species. As many as 50 million Americans are lactose intolerant and cannot digest dairy products. The insistence that milk calcium is crucial to the maintenance of our bones can be questioned ... the bioavailability of milk calcium may not be as good as other calcium compounds, and milk lacks other minerals and vitamins important to bone maintenance. Why, it can be asked, do the human populations that consume the most cow's milk have the highest rates of osteoporosis. Milk is seriously lacking in several other critically essential nutrients. Many consumers do not want to drink milk that comes from cows that are treated with anti-biotics and recombinant bovine growth hormone (rBGH), and argue that labeling should indicate whether or not the milk or dairy products come from treated cows. New arguments are emerging that question the need for dairy calcium for bone health. Credible research identifies strong associations with allergies, inflammatory responses, and some chronic disease. The seriousness and high prevalence of lactose intolerance may not be exaggerated, and may be a major concern for a substantial portion of the global population.

The Ugly

Cow's milk can be separated into two main types: type A1 and type A2. New evidence has recently been uncovered to identify an opiate substance in A1 milk, dubbed BCM-7, that is directly linked with diabetes, heart disease, schizophrenia, autism, and sudden-death-syndrome. Mechanisms have been identified. The credibility of the research and findings is very high.

Conclusions, implications, and call for action

The issues identified in Chapter Three are enough to cause genuine concern, but *if* the evidence regarding the BCM-7 molecule is credible, then the seriousness of the implications are even more alarming, and warrant a call for responsibility ... and action.

A note about understanding the scientific method, the use of biostatistics, and causality

Reading and trying to understand scientific literature can often be mind-boggling. Not only do scientists and academics speak in a language riddled with subject-specific terminology, but they converse using a host of specialized concepts. Without at least a rudimentary understanding of these basic concepts, it is difficult to follow their reasoning and to understand the information offered. This is especially true in the general field of human biology, because our physiology is so fantastically complicated, things normally happen on such a minuscule scale, and very often incredibly fast.

I once read that a major difference between Chinese medicine and Western medicine was that the Chinese were bound by cultural restraints prohibiting them from dissecting human bodies and organs, while westerners were not shy about chopping up human corpses to see first-hand what was going on. This implied that the Chinese could only analyze and attempt to understand biological phenomena via observation of the body as a whole, whereas western scientists could dissect and isolate and thereby get down to the nitty-gritty.

But this difference is only partly true. Our biochemistry and physiological activity is so intrinsic, so complicated, so microscopic, and often so quick, that we westerners are often obligated to view 'only at a distance' as well. This is why a great deal of human biological science is achieved by studying populations, or 'epidemiology'. Through studying selected populations, or groups of people, we can observe the occurrence of disease or certain characteristics ... and we can use numbers ... 'statistics' ... to try to give these observations meaning. Words, or concepts, like 'prevalence' and 'incidence' are applied to give us a picture of how many within the population are affected, and to what degree. By analyzing the numbers we can determine degrees of 'association' and 'correlation'. With these statistical tools we try to predict outcomes, applying a measure of 'probability'. We can then say that such and such a condition is 'associated' with another. Using a word that implies more credibility, we can go a step further and say that one phenomenon is 'linked' to another. The end goal becomes that of establishing a 'causal' relationship ... the familiar 'cause-and-effect' scenario ... where one thing *causes* another.

The more that is known about an association or linkage, the stronger the connection, and the greater the credibility. A key measure of the strength of the connection is the correlation. The more closely that the occurrence of one condition 'fits' with another, the higher the correlation. A 100% occurrence of one phenomenon with another would calculate to a correlation of 1.0, while a total lack of mutual occurrence would result in a 0.0 correlation.

These concepts are especially useful in understanding the association and linkage of the consumption of cow's milk with health affects and disease conditions.

Another key element in establishing credible associations and linkages is the ability to identify a verifiable biological 'mechanism'. Deriving a number, or a correlation, is one thing, but to be able to explain an actual mechanism puts us leap-jumps ahead. This is an important part of the recent research re the BCM-7 molecule, and its link with disease conditions.

Going one step further, the association or linkage gains its final status of credibility if 'causation' can be established. But causality in itself is a very evasive thing. You may have heard the statements "association does not prove causation" or "correlation does not imply causation" or that "true causality is impossible to prove". These conclusions are a part of every beginning course in statistics. However, popular writings about nutrition, health, and medicine are riddled with claims or implications of causality. Much of your doctors convincing statements are based on claims or implications of causality.

My favorite example, and a major pet-peeve, is the implication that cholesterol *causes* the build-up of plaque in your arteries, or the condition named 'atherosclerosis'. We are constantly being bombarded with warnings about consuming high cholesterol foods, and everyone at any risk at all for hypertension, heart disease, or stroke, is strongly advised by their doctor to lower their cholesterol. But scientific research has made it clear for some time now that (1) the body produces its own cholesterol, and diet cholesterol has a very weak association with plaque build-up, and that (2) the body's activity to create plague build-up is known to be a response to an earlier 'incident' at the arterial wall ... or, in other words, the body is trying to *repair* a weak or damaged arterial wall. The conclusion is then (3) that cholesterol is the *material* used by the body to make a repair, but is *not* the *cause* of the effort to do so.

It is true that lowering *body* cholesterol will decrease plaque build-up, simply because you are depriving the body of the material to build with. But in medical research and inquiry, little has been directed to studying the source of the problem ... attempting to answer *why* the arterial wall is

11

weak or damaged and needs repair in the first place. A few maverick studies suggest that the problem is nutritional. More about this in another part of the series, *The Nutrition Factor: A Bold New Perspective*.

Your doctor is fond of prescribing Lipitor to lower body cholesterol, and of course he gets his usual pharmaceutical cut. Lipitor has been the top-selling drug in the world for several years now, with profits in the billions, with its competitor, Zocor, running a close second place.

Another important concept in understanding statistics, and especially the cause and effect relationship, is the interference of *confounders*. A strong correlation may exist between, say, A and B, such as we are tempted to say that A causes B, or B causes A ... but it may be possible that something separate from both of them is the cause ... C may be the cause of both A and B, or either of them. 'C' is then a potential confounder. This is an important issue in understanding the relationship between calcium and bone health, and the disease condition, osteoporosis.

Types of research studies and the problem of bias.

A common core requirement within the curriculum for a master's degree in the natural sciences is learning how to critically analyze research studies and scientific literature. This is an essential and very valuable skill to master, because scientific studies may be poorly designed, with possible procedural and logical errors, with unintentional or even intentional bias, and authoritative statements can be based on misinformation or on an arbitrary point of view. It is unfortunate, but many of the presumed experts in a particular field, and even the scientists themselves, have by-passed this critical part of their education. These can include medical doctors, whose pre-med and medical school training did not include this skill-learning in their curriculums, and also includes self-proclaimed experts whose background did not encompass a rigorous master's degree curriculum.

When critiquing a given study or writing, the most common errors are bias, poor study design and methodology, misinformation, and illogical conclusions.

Bias, or 'non-objectivity', can result from a number of factors and influences, and can be truly unintentional, or can be purposefully included. The type of bias which much of my writing in *The Nutrition Factor: A Bold New Perspective* is directed against, is that derived from the scientist's own prejudiced point of view. The Germans have an excellent word to describe this 'point of view' concept more broadly, namely the word *weltanschauung,* which literally translated means "world view". However, weltanschauung is ones world view in a very broad sense, including an individual's religion and philosophy, their ethnocentrism and cultural base, and everything that comes together to describe their total view of the world. A less-broad word for this is one's *paradigm.* This world view ... or weltanschauung, or paradigm ... is the aura from within which every scientist begins his enquiry, and can profoundly affect the design, method, results, and conclusions of a study, often totally unintentionally or occurring without those being involved truly understanding that it is happening.

Unfortunately, bias can also be the result of mischievous and purposeful manipulation. One sees this most often when (a) a study is funded and/or directed by a special interest group (i.e. the dairy industry), or (b) when a study is intended to support a pre-determined conclusion and/or result (i.e. the dairy industry, again), and (c) when a study is overtly influenced by a religious or cultural belief (i.e. vegetarianism).

Or, bias can simply be wrong conclusions founded on misinformation or illogical reasoning.

However, a great deal of bias can be the result of poor study design and methodology. It is here that the reader or student can most effectively employ his critiquing skills.

The study of individuals or populations to obtain information about their physical status or health can be most simply divided into the following four methodologies:

1. Screening ... Used to separate those with a probability or risk of having a certain disease condition from a larger population of apparently healthy individuals. The target condition must be identifiable and a reliable test available to detect that condition.

2. Sampling ... Used to obtain information about a large population by testing a sample of the population. The term 'random sampling' refers to the method of sampling or the choosing of test subjects by which no pre-determined pattern or knowledge of who is to be selected is known.

Another variation of sampling is a 'cross-sectional study', which is used to measure the prevalence of a targeted condition within a population. It should be noted that because the whole population is not surveyed, cross-sectional analysis does not determine the 'incidence' of the condition, only prevalence.

4. Observation Studies ... Observational studies are the most common of all scientific studies ... a condition is simply observed under different conditions or different time periods. The investigator has no control of the input or outcome … he or she engages in no or very little intervention.

The usual purpose of observation studies is to determine the *etiology*, or cause, of a condition (i.e. disease condition). However, true causation is seldom achieved, and investigators instead determine the relative strength of 'associations' or 'linkages'/

Observational studies can be sub-divided as follows:

(a) Case-Control, or Retrospective Studies … The investigator makes an observation regarding the possible cause of a particular condition evidenced currently or retrospectively within a population, forms a hypothesis to explain the association, and then tests the hypothesis. In a case-control study all of the relevant events (i.e. disease and exposure) have already occurred when the study is started. The study goes back in time to the past (i.e. from disease to exposure). The incidence and prevalence of the condition is measured. Statistical analysis is usually employed to then determine correlation and probability.

(b) Cohort, or Prospective Studies … Four different descriptive terms are used for prospective studies: *cohort, incidence, prospective,* and *longitudinal.* Cohort refers to the study group … cohorts, or a group of individuals sharing a common factor. Incidence is the measure of the number or percentage of the individuals within the population which have the target condition. Prospective means that the study group is followed forward in time to the future (i.e. from exposure to disease).

The investigator typically assembles a group of volunteers (cohort) and examines them to make certain they are free of the condition (i.e. disease) in question at the start of the study. Numerous items of information are collected. The cohort is then kept under sufficient observation to identify those who develop the condition that is under study. A *control group*, or a similar group of individuals who are *not* exposed to the hypothetical cause of the condition, is often formed as a base for comparison.

The cohort design, by its very nature, avoids two of the most potent causes of bias in the retrospective approach, namely the selection of controls and possible bias in determining exposure. The cohort design is therefore considered to be more rigorous and credible.

One of the major limitations of the cohort approach stems from the fact that participants are usually volunteers who must return at regular intervals to be examined for development of the targeted condition, and there is limited control of other outside factors that the participants may be exposed to, and which can potentially affect the outcome.

However, the different study designs are not necessarily competing methods. Clinical observation or a prevalence survey (a cross-sectional study) may provide the first suggestion of an association, which can then be tested via a retrospective study. If the suspected association is confirmed, a cohort prospective study can be a third step.

5. **Experimental Studies** ... Obsevational studies in which the investigator has 'control' of the input ... intervention is usually a part of the study. The purpose of experimental studies are usually *not* to determine cause or the strength of associations, but instead are to determine which is the superior or more effective treatment to correct a condition (i.e. disease condition).

The experiment is the strongest weapon in the scientific armament to test a theoretical association or suspected cause-and-effect relationship

The hallmark of experimental interventions is the random allocation of subjects to various treatment groups ... each group is treated differently, and everything is as randomized as possible. This is the **randomized clinical trial** method.

As with observational cohort studies, clinical trials are prospective, in that the study is carried forward in time.

Potential bias due to the expectations of the subjects is commonly minimized by not only randomizing the treatment , but by also designing the study so that the subjects do not know which treatment they are receiving. This also minimizes the *placebo effect*, or a false change in condition caused by the expectations of the treated subject. Bias due to the expectations of the investigators themselves can be minimized by employing the technique of 'double blinding' where both the investigator and the subject do not know which treatment the participants are being subjected to.

It is essential in randomized clinical trials that *all* participants are analyzed ... this is considered to be the 'golden rule' of randomized clinical trials. If only some of the subjects are analyzed, the credibility of the results and conclusions is seriously impeded.

A note about the RDAs and DRIs

The RDAs, or Recommended Dietary Allowances are defined as "the levels of intake of essential nutrients that, on the basis of scientific knowledge, are judged by the Food and Nutrition Board to be adequate to meet the known nutrient needs of practically all healthy person" (RDA,

1989). The intakes recommended are based on the observed mean (average) requirements, taken from scientific studies, and adjusted to cover the needs of 97.7% of the population. The RDAs have been reviewed and adjusted approximately every ten years, beginning in 1941. Research carried out for determining the RDAs was exhaustive and thorough, and one cannot help but deeply respect the work that went into each report's compilation.

Beginning in 1997, the Food and Nutrition Board (FNB) of the Institute of Medicine (IOM) published a series of DRIs, or *Dietary Reference Intakes* to replace the former RDAs, and were "developed in recognition of the growing and diverse uses of quantitative reference values and the availability of more sophisticated approaches for dietary planning and assessment purposes" (Dietary Reference Intakes, 2006, preface).

However, the effort was carried out 'within the framework of the conventional wisdom', and I, for one, have always questioned their results, and wondered what was their thoughts supporting their outcomes. I would like to take the case of vitamin C as an example. We know that we only need as little as 13 milligrams of vitamin C per day to ward off the overt symptoms of the deficiency condition known as 'scurvy'. Yet vitamin C is essential for many other body functions, such as (a) the biosynthesis of carnitine, which is essential in the transport of fatty acids into the mitochondria of cells, (b) is required to sustain the activity of the copper-containing enzyme *dopamine oxygenase*, which catalyzes the oxidation of dopamine to form the neurotransmitter norepinephrine, (c) is involved in the degradation of the amino acid tyrosine, (d) is the reducing agent for the activation of several hormones, (e) is required for the optimal activity of various drug-destroying metabolic systems, (f) it is considered a powerful antioxidant, (g) it facilitates the absorption and transfer of iron and calcium, (h) it assists in the conversion of the inactive form of the vitamin folic acid into its active form, dihydrofolic acid and tetrahydrofolic acid, (i) plays a role in alleviating allergic reactions, enhancing immune function, stimulating the formation of bile, and facilitating the release of some steroid hormones, (j) is necessary for the conversion of cholesterol to bile acids, and (k), is reported to be involved in the detoxification of many chemical carcinogens.

Its *most* notable function, however, is the critical role that it takes in the formation of the protein *collagen*. Collagen is the major structural protein of bodily connective tissue, binding cells and tissues together in bone, teeth, cartilage, skin, scar tissue *and the walls of your arteries and capillaries*. Vitamin C is specifically required by the *fibroblast* cells of connective tissue, *and the bone-forming osteoblasts within bone.* Any deficiency in vitamin C results in defective collagen synthesis, and is evidenced by impaired wound healing, disruption of capillaries, and faulty bone and teeth formation. One of the first effects of any impairment of collagen synthesis are small pinpoint hemorrhages, which result from weakness in the membranes that line the blood capillaries and in the fibers that hold cells together under the surface of the skin. The involvement of vitamin C in collagen formation during scar tissue formation has led some researchers to suggest that vitamin C intake should be increased to *50 times the RDA* both before and after surgery. (Human Nutrition, pp 438-50).

The RDA for vitamin C in the 1989 10th Edition was set at 60 milligrams. I noted that this was the amount found in one tall glass of orange juice, or in one good-sized whole orange, or in three large strawberries. So it would seem to be rather easy to obtain in a diet 'consuming a variety of basic foods and maintaining a balanced diet'. But there has been much debate on how much our RDA for this vitamin should *really* be. During the 90's this debate raged ... some saying it should be 500 mg, others saying even more. The most conservative were suggesting that 225 would be reasonable. The famous scientist, Dr. Linus Pauling, insisted that we needed much, much more ... and in his own life he consumed 18 grams (18,000 milligrams) of ascorbic acid every day for the last 25 years of his life, finally passing away at the age of 93.

Now ... obtaining 60 mg of vitamin C every day, as I stated, would be relatively easy. But 500 mg ?? .... or even 225 mg ?? This would be a different matter, indeed. Even at 225 mg, this would mean ingesting almost 4 tall glasses of orange juice, or 4 large oranges, or 11 large strawberries. And because vitamin C is a water-soluble vitamin, and conventional wisdom states that an excess of this vitamin is quickly removed in the urine, we must have that intake on a daily basis ... *each* and *every* day ... no allowance for having more one day and storing the excess, and then having less another day, and making use of the stored excess. One then is prompted to ask the question: "Does the availability in normal foods have anything to do with the determination of the RDAs?"

I was enrolled at the University of Hawaii at the time I was studying the RDAs, and wondering about this question, and so I made a phone call to one of the Food and Nutrition Board members, who was then attached to the Cancer Research Center in Honolulu, and I asked the question. He was very amiable, and was delighted that I had called him and asked this question. He laughed and answered: "No ... we consider the scientific evidence for the need, not the availability in food."

But I still wonder. The current RDA/AI for vitamin C has been increased, and is separated as follows: Infants 0-6 months, 40 mg; 7-12 months, 50 mg; children 1-3 years 15 mg, 4-6 years 25 mg; males and females 9-13 years 45 mg; females 14-18 yrs 65 mg, males 14-18 years and females 19 years and over, 75 mg; pregnant women 18 years or younger, 80 mg; pregnant women over 18, 85 mg; lactating women 18 or younger, 115 mg; and lactating women over 18, 120 mg. (USDA, Dietary Reference Intakes, current) It is significant that infants up to one year are thought to need 40-50 milligrams of vitamin C ... I will refer to this again in Chapter Three.

In response to important findings in nutritional research, plus the recognition that the RDAs did not address the varied requirements of different individuals, the Food and Nutrition Board, now under the auspices of the Institute of Medicine, The National Academies, began an initiative to develop a new set of values known as the DRIs, or Dietary Reference Intakes. Included in this new set of values are the AIs, or 'Adequate Intakes', and the ULs, or 'Upper Limits' of intake (*The Development of DRIs, 2008*). The values in this book are taken from the most current update of these references, available from the USDA Food and Nutrition Information Center, Dietary Reference Intakes, readily accessible online at www.fnic.nal.usda.gov/nal

A note about measurements

For those of you not familiar with common measurements in nutrition, and conversions back and forth with the metric system, here are a few tips:

Measurements of nutrient amounts can be confusing. The milligram, abbreviated to 'mg' is the most common form of measurement for nutrients, which is $1/1000^{th}$ of a gram (g). And 28.35 grams equal one ounce (oz). Going up in scale, one thousand grams is a kilogram (kg), which is equal to 2.21 pounds (lbs). Going smaller, $1/1000^{th}$ of a milligram is called a microgram (mcg), which can also be written as 'μg'. The preferred unit for measuring vitamin A is the RAE, which is the 'retinol activity equivalent', and which is considered to be the same as a microgram (mcg, or μg). Liquid measurements are also used. A liter is 1.06 U.S. quarts, one fluid ounce equals 29.57 mililiters. An 8 ounce serving of milk is 236.58 militers, or 0.237 liters, or 244.2 grams (average specific gravity of milk is 1.032).

The term 'calorie' is actually a misnomer … the correct term is the *kilocalorie*, which is defined as the amount of heat energy required to raise the temperature of one kilogram of water one degree centigrade at normal atmospheric pressure (the atmospheric pressure at sea level). 'Kilocalorie' can be abbreviated to 'kcalorie' or 'kcal', or is often written as 'Calorie' (with a capital 'C')

References used in the text for Chapter One

Guthrie, Helen A.; Picciano, Mary Frances; *Human Nutrition*, Mosby-Year Book, Inc., 1995. This is a marvelous text book, used by countless university nutrition classes throughout the U.S. and world.

Institute of Medicine, *The Development of DRIs, 1994 – 2004, Lessons Learned and New Challenges*, The National Academies Press, 2008.

Institute of Medicine, *Dietary Reference Intakes, The Essential Guide to Nutrient Requirements*, The National Academies Press, 2006.

International Livestock Research Institute, *Milk chemistry – An introductrion.*www.ilri.org/infoserv/webpub/fulldocs/ilca_manual4/Milkchemistr

National Research Council; *Recommeded Dietary Allowance,10th Edition,* Subcommittee on the Tenth Edition of the RDAs, Food and Nutrition Board, National Academy Press, 1989

USDA, *Dietary Reference Intakes*, Nutritional Information Center, www.fnic.nal.usda.gov/nal

USDA, *National Nutrient Data base for Standard Reference,* Nutrient Data Laboratory, Agricultural Research Service, www.nal.usda.gov/fnic/foodcomp

Wade, Nicholas; *Lactose Tolerance in East Africa Points to Recent Evolution,* The New York Times, December 11, 2006.

Wikipedia, *Milk*, www.en.wikipedia.org/wiki/Milk

CHAPTER TWO

'THE GOOD'

An important food choice

A single eight-ounce glass of whole milk provides an American adult 14% of their recommended protein intake with 139 kcalories of energy, 25.6% of their daily need for calcium, 27.2 % of their required phosphorous, 31.9% of the B-vitamin, riboflavin, 13.1% of vitamin A, 42.6 % of B-12, 16.9% B-6, and 12.6 % of their omega-3 requirement. (USDA, IOM).

There is no question that milk *can* be a very important source of many of the nutrients that our bodies need. From this simple summary of the nutrient benefits, one cannot help but conclude that all the hype and enthusiasm that every one of us has heard since our toddler days about the goodness of milk and the need to drink several glasses every day is fully justified.

Consumption and availability

And yes, we *do* consume a lot of milk and other dairy products. Although we did not domesticate the cow sufficiently to extract milk from its udder for our own consumption until perhaps 7,000 years ago, cow's milk has become a major food choice worldwide. Northern Europeans consume the highest per capita amounts, with Finland topping the list at 183.9 liters of liquid milk per person per annum, 19.1 kilograms of cheese, and 5.3 kilograms of butter. Due to population size, however, the U.S. produces the largest amount of cow's milk, with total tonnage reaching 82.5 million tons in 2006 (University of Guelph, 2010).

The case of India

In the country of India the cow is deeply revered as a sacred animal, and its milk is thought to be "the best of all nutritive substances ... literally life-giving". (Godbole, 2007, pp 5)

Many references to the value and importance of milk are included in the *Vedas*, considered to be the oldest books in the world, and the *Aryrveda*, which is the ancient Medical Sciences of the Hindus. An example of the writings is as follows:

"And since milk is kindred in its nature to the essential principles of life and so very congenial to the panzoism of all created animals, its use may be unreservedly recommended to all and is not forbidden in diseases due to the deranged action of Vayu or Pittam or in ailments affecting the mind or the vascular system of man. Its beneficial and curative efficacy may be witnessed in cases of chronic fever, in cough, dyspepsia, phthisis and other wasting diseases, in Gulma (abdominal glands), insanity, ascites, epileptic fits, in vertigo, in delirium, in burning sensation of the body, in thirst, in diseases affecting the heart and the bladder, in chlorosis and dysentery, in piles, colic and obstinate constipation, in Grahani, Pravahika, miscarriage and other diseases peculiar to the female reproductive organs, and in haemoptysis. It is a refrigerant and acts as a bracing beverage after physical exercise. It is sacred, constructive, tonic, spermatopoietic, rejuvenating and aphrodisiac. It expands the intellectual capacities of a man, brings about the adhesion of broken or fractured bones, rejuvenates used and exhausted frames, forms an excellent enemata, increases the duration of life and acts as a vitalizer. It is an emetic and purgative remedy and imparts a healthy rotundity to the frame and which through its kindred or similar properties augments the quality of bodily albumen and is the most complete and wholesome diet for infants, old men and persons suffering from cachexia witnessed in cases of ulcers in the chest, as well as for persons debilitated from insufficient food, sexual excesses or excessive physical labor." (Godbole, 2007, pp 5)

Beginning in the year 2001 India surpassed the U.S. in total amount of animal milk production … which includes that from the water buffalo … reaching just under 100 million tons in 2006. (U of Guelph and Wikipedia, including buffalo milk production).

Calcium, vitamin D, lactose … and human evolution

Cow's milk contains a great deal of calcium, and is a prime source for this critically essential minera. Plus, cow's milk is uniquely formulated to maximize the absorption of calcium by the human body, especially if it is fortified with vitamin D.

Estimations of how much Americans actually rely on milk and milk products for their calcium intake vary, ranging from 42% (Cook, 2003), 45% (More, 2008), 70% (Gue´guen, 2000) to as much as 73% (International Dairy Foods Association, 2009). The current U.S. RDA/DRIs for calcium is 40-50 milligrams for infants, 500-600 mg for young children, 1,000 mg per day for adults, and 1,300 milligrams for adolescents and pregnant or lactating mothers. An 8-ounce glass of cow's milk contains 257 mg of calcium. (USDA, NDB No. 01211)

It may be prudent to introduce one different perspective of our need for calcium at this point, which will re-surface in the next chapter. This is the calcium intake consumed by earlier man, as explained by one of the pioneers in this exciting new field of study, S. Boyd Eaton. He suggests the following:

> "The nutritional requirements of contemporary humans were almost certainly established over eons of evolutionary experience and the best available evidence indicates that this evolution occurred in a high-calcium nutritional environment. The exercise and dietary patterns of humans living at the end of the Stone Age can be considered natural paradigms: calcium intake was twice that for contemporary humans and requirements for physical exertion were also greater than at present. Bony remains from that period suggest that Stone Agers developed a greater peak bone mass and experienced less age-related bone loss than do humans in the 20th Century." (Eaton, 1991)

Although the role of calcium is commonly thought to be mostly with bone formation and maintenance, it's more important function in terms of overall human physiology is its involvement as a cofactor in numerous other-than-bone biochemical pathways. Only 1% of body calcium is used in outside bone metabolism, and the blood concentration of calcium is only 0.0001 part of the blood mass, its blood concentration is tightly controlled by automatic regulatory control, or *homeostasis*. The bone is actually used by the body as a storage site for calcium, and calcium is withdrawn or added as needed. Examples of the non-bone roles of calcium include (a) synapses reactions in the contraction of muscle fibers, (b) functioning as a catalyst in the formation of fibrin, which is essential in blood clotting, (c) initiating neurotransmitter release in the nervous system, (d) involvement in the absorption of vitamin B12, (e) as a catalyst in the formation of the fat-digesting enzyme 'pancreatic lipase', and (f) its role in the secretion of insulin from the pancreas. There are many more such functions ... these are only a few of the most well-known.

In contrast to common thinking, bone is not a solid, relatively fixed mass, but is a living, constantly changing organism, and is very complex in its make-up and metabolism. We have yet to fully understand the intricacies of how bone is both constructed or resorbed (absorbed *again*). But we do know a great deal. Bone is 60 to 66% mineral, by weight, which is mainly hydroxyapatite and calcium phosphate, with the remaining 34 to 40% water and protein. Hydroxyapatite (Ca_{10} [PO_4]$_6$ [OH]$_2$) and calcium phosphate are mostly calcium and phosphate, in an approximate ratio of 2:1.

Bone is constantly being made and resorbed, which continues throughout one's life. The main structural bone cells are the 'osteoblasts', which secrete collagen to form a basic matrix, which is then filled and mineralized by calcium and phosphorous. The break-down and resorption of previously made bone is carried out by the 'osteoclast' cells, the activity of which is regulated by a number of hormones. Skeletal turnover in children and adolescents occurs so that that formation of bone exceeds resorption, thus contributing to bone growth. This excess of formation over resorption continues into adulthood until peak mass is obtained at some point between the ages of 30 and 40. It is thought that bone mass density steadily declines after reaching its peak, continuing to decline throughout the rest of one's life, although the rate of decline can be influenced by the intake of the minerals and vitamins involved in bone formation, and other factors. The condition observed when the bone density declines to the point of making the bone structurally weak is termed 'osteoporosis'.

It should be noted that essential nutrients necessary for bone metabolism include many other minerals, such as magnesium, zinc, sodium, fluoride, manganese, iron, iodine, cobalt, molybdenum, vanadium, silicon, and boron. Vitamins involved include vitamins A, B-6 and B-12, and vitamins C and D and K. Hormones associated with bone maintenance include the sex hormones estrogen and testosterone; human growth hormone (hGH); insulin, produced by the pancreas beta cells; tri-iodothyronine (T_3) and tetraiodothyronine (T_4), produced by the thyroid gland; parathyroid, secreted by the parathyroid glands; and calcitonin, also secreted by the thyroid gland.

(Sources for the information in the previous four paragraphs are the textbooks *Human Nutrition* by Guthrie and Picciano, *Advanced Nutrition and Human Metabolism* by Groff, Gropper, and Hunt; and *Principles of Anatomy and Physiology, Seventh Edition* by Tortora and Grabowski.)

This summary illustrates the importance of the minerals and vitamins critical to bone construction and maintenance, all of which are supplied by cow's milk. The most critical are calcium and phosphorous. However, because phosphorous is amply supplied in our diet without the consumption of milk and milk products, whereas calcium is much more difficult to obtain in sufficient quantity and bioavailability from other sources, the main focus turns to calcium.

Cow's milk as a source for calcium is especially suited for consumption by humans because it contains substances that significantly enhance the absorption of calcium. This has been a controversial and much-studied phenomenon, and not all the mechanisms are fully understood. One particular review of interest is that by Leon Geuguen et al (the term 'et al' meaning 'group' or 'team') entitled *The Bioavailability of Dietary Calcium* (Gueguen, 2000). In the section of this excellent article, entitled *Peculiarities and advantages of the calcium in milk and dairy products,* he concludes that: "the calcium in milk differs in several interesting features from the calcium in other foodstuffs or supplements" … "Because it is bound to peptides and proteins, milk calcium is more likely to remain in a solution" … "Milk calcium may be absorbed in the absence of vitamin D, under the influence of lactose in the distal small intestine via the paracellular route. Thus milk can provide calcium with 'ensured absorbability' which is generally insensitive to external factors" … "Dairy products do not contain anything likely to inhibit the intestinal absorption of calcium, like phytates, oxalates, uronic acids or the polyphenols of certain plant foods" … "These advantages cannot be provided by any other source of calcium" … "As milk provides calcium with 'protected absorbability', 'prolonged absorption' and 'extended bone deposition', milk is the most suitable dietary constituent that meets the high calcium intake required …".

Marvin Harris, in his engrossing book, *Good to Eat, Riddles of Food and Culture*, relates the fascinating story of how the need for calcium shaped the peoples of northern Europe's evolutionary path, favoring the domestication of the cow for its milk, and lighter colored skin to increase the availability of vitamin D. Cultural anthropologists explain that, as human populations moved out of Africa, they encountered a number of challenges for their food supply and nutrition. A shortage of vitamin C, and resulting scurvy, was surely one of them. But here the milk of animals could not help, because their milk contained little of this vitamin … they produce their own vitamin C and do not need to acquire it in their mother's milk. Calcium was another nutrient that became in short supply, as humans left their jungle environment behind, and green leafy plants became scarcer. This was particularly the case when humans travelled north to lands that were heavily forested, and which characterized long harsh winters. In this new environment there was little opportunity to seek out or nurture the sort of vegetation that was rich in calcium, and coupled with the low relative bioavailability of calcium from leafy plants, finding sources of calcium thus became a life-threatening issue.

A lack of calcium causes the disease condition named 'rickets', which is evidenced by poor bone formation, considerable structural deformity, and a short stature. The presence of rickets was clearly a strong negative factor for natural selection among earlier human populations. Individuals with rickets were fragile, small, and did not survive well. Babies were small, unhealthy, and often deformed; and the female pelvises of the rickets victims were small and misshaped, and these mothers could not deliver babies well.

All mammal mothers, including humans, produce milk for their babies, and all of these variations of mother's milk contain the complex sugar *lactose*. In order to digest and utilize the lactose, all animal babies possess the ability to produce the enzyme *lactase*. However, animal infants universally lose this function after weaning … in each animal species, including us humans … at least, that is, without genetic or phenotype alteration. It is theorized that the first European humans to acquire the genetic modification to become lactase sufficient after infancy, and were therefore able to digest lactose into adulthood, were the members of the Funnel Beaker Culture of northern Europe, who raised cattle and consumed the milk from their udders earlier than other groups. This ability to utilize animal milk greatly enhanced the potential for these people to better survive, and gave individuals who had the capability to drink animal milk a great advantage.

But it was crucial that these early northern Europeans not only be able to drink milk, but that they could also efficiently absorb its nutrients. Again, calcium was one nutrient most in need. However, the absorption of calcium is influenced by a variety of factors, the most important of which is the availability of vitamin D. Plus lactose, the main sugar in milk.

Almost no calcium can be absorbed without vitamin D, except with high amounts of lactose. Now, the origin of vitamin D is from sunlight, either absorbed directly, or as 'cholecalciferol' (vitamin D_3) acquired from the flesh of animals which have previously synthesized the vitamin from sunlight. When the skin of humans or animals is exposed to ultraviolet radiation (sunlight), 7-dehydrocholesterol within the skin is converted into a compound known as 'provitamin D_3'. It is known that low levels of sunlight will inhibit the amount of the provitamin synthesized. For example, the amount of sunshine available during the months of November through February at a latitude equivalent to the city of Boston

25

is insufficient to produce significant vitamin D synthesis (Human Nutrition, pp 415).

The efficiency of our human skin to synthesize vitamin D is also dependent on the amount of pigmentation, or 'melanin' in the skin … the pigmentation blocks ultra-violet radiation …and dark-skinned people therefore produce less vitamin D with equivalent sunlight. As an observed consequence, modern-age darker-skinned individuals living in northern cities are at particular risk for vitamin D deficiency.

Harris brings all these factors together in his delightful narrative to explain how the need for calcium led the peoples of northern Europe to seek the milk of the cow as a food choice, and to develop light-colored skin in order to maximize vitamin D synthesis.

Use of cow's milk as a food was therefore a major factor in the survival, expansion, and evolution of earlier human populations. Studies by Dr. Sarah Tishkoff and her team from the University of Maryland, have shown that as many as three separate groups in early East Africa independently acquired the genetic base for adult lactase sufficiency as early as 7,000 years ago. Their investigations suggest that these groups were able to survive and increase their population by a factor as much as ten times that compared to groups who were not lactase sufficient and did not consume cow's milk.

Calcium and hypertension

It has been shown for some time now, through a large number of studies, that calcium deficiency is linked to hypertension. This was first recognized in the 1970s when it was discovered that communities drinking 'hard water' … water that has a high concentration of calcium … had significantly lower death rates from cardiovascular disease. The association, however, is not consistent among different individuals. Some persons are more 'calcium sensitive' than others, meaning that the high blood pressure condition in some persons is more responsive to additional intakes of calcium than others. It also has been found that systolic blood pressure is more affected than diastolic, and that there is often a threshold level of intake. Calcium intakes of more than 800 mg per day are required in order to affect hypertension. (*Advanced Nutrition and Human Metabolism, 2000*)

Protein ... casein, whey .... quality of

As stated at the beginning of this chapter, an 8-ounce serving of cow's milk provides 7.2 grams of protein, which fulfills about 14% of our RDA for adults. Four glasses would give us about 29 grams, which would equal 56% of our RDA. All of this with only 550 kcalories if whole milk was the milk of choice, or only 381 kcalories if it was lowfat milk.

A quick trip to your closest health food store would reveal that there are a large number of products for sale utilizing the casein or whey proteins from milk, extolling the benefits and advantages of these two proteins. They are very popular among body-builders. Casein is known to be a 'slow' protein, digesting slowly and thoroughly, and protecting the body from muscle protein breakdown, or 'catabolism'. Whey, on the other hand, is known to be a 'fast' protein', being picked up by body cells and used to build needed body proteins quickly ... within less than one hour after intake. The whey products are very popular sellers ... you could even say that there is a current 'fad' favoring the use of whey protein ... many consider whey protein to be the 'ultimate' in available food proteins, because it is a 'complete' protein, meaning that it contains all of the 9 *essential* amino acids, and is rich in all of them.

There are several methods to determine and compare the *quality* of proteins. 'Quality' can be interpreted in different ways, and can include the concepts of bioavailability, the amino acid composition (chemical score), a measure of the nitrogen balance (biological value), net protein utilization, and the contribution to weight gain. However, in 1993 the US Food and Drug Administration (FDA) and the Food and Agricultural Organization of the United Nations (FAO/WHO) adopted the *Protein Digestibility Corrected Amino Acid Score* (PDCAAS) as 'the preferred best' method to determine protein quality. This method gives milk (and egg) protein the highest ranking value. Milk proteins are thus considered to be the best quality among all the food sources. A list of food sources for protein with their rating on a zero to 1.00 scale is as follows:

Milk	1.00	Fruits	0.76
Egg	1.00	Vegetables	0.73
Beef	0.92	Legumes	0.70
Soybean	0.91	Cereals	0.59
Chickpeas	0.78	Whole Wheat	0.42

It can be credibly argued, then, that cow's milk is the *best* food source for the protein that our bodies require.

Minerals

The USDA Food Composition Data Base lists data for a total of 10 minerals ... *all of which are contained in cow's milk*. The following table list the minerals, the content per 8-ounce serving of milk, the RDA for that mineral, and the percent RDA that this serving supplies.

Mineral	Amount Per 8-oz serving	RDA	% RDA in serving
Calcium (mg)	256.5	1,000	25.6
Iron (mg)	0.03	13.0	1.52
Magnesium (mg)	22.7	370	4.14
Phosphorous (mg)	190.7	700	27.2
Potassium (mg)	299.6	4,700	4.37
Sodium (mg)	97.6	1,500	4.5
Zinc (mg)	0.84	9.5	8.8
Copper (mcg)	56.8	900	4.3
Manganese (mg)	0.009	2.05	1.44
Selenium (mcg)	6.81	55	14.4

(USDA, NDB No. 01211)

Vitamins

Food composition analysis has been completed by the USDA for all of the known 14 essential vitamins except the B-vitamin, biotin. Data for these 13 vitamins is also included in the NDB No. 01211 summary for whole milk. Cow's milk is shown to contain all of the 13 vitamins except vitamin C. The following table outlines this data, again based on a single 8-ounce serving.

Vitamin	Amount Per 8-oz serving	RDA	% RDA in serving
Vitamin C (mg)	0	82.5	0
Thiamin (mg)	0.104	1.15	9.1
Riboflavin (mg)	0.384	1.2	31.9
Niacin (mg)	0.202	15	1.35
Pantothenic acid (mg)	0.847	5	16.9
Vitamin B-6 (mg)	0.082	1.3	4.3
Folate (mcg)	11.35	400	2.84
Choline (mg)	32.5	487.5	4.66
Vitamin B-12 (mcg)	1.022	2.4	42.6
Vitamin A (RAE, mcg)	104.4	800	13.05
Vitamin E (mg)	0.159	15	1.06
Vitamin D (mcg)	0.227	0.1	4.54
Vitamin K (mcg)	0.681	105	1.65

This shows that cow's milk contains all of the essential vitamins except vitamin C and possibly biotin.

Essential fatty acids

I am sure you have heard about omega-6 and omega-3 … or *linoleic acid* and *linolenic acid*. These are the two types of fat that are *essential* to our body's functioning … in other words, we *cannot do without them in our diet*. These two fats are classified as *polyunsatuarated* fats, and their metabolism leads to a host of very critical pathways.

Omega-6 is fairly common in our normal food supply, especially since the 'fat revolution' of the 50's and early 60's when Americans turned to vegetable oils and away from saturated fats, particularly butter. Almost all vegetable oils are rich in omega-6, or linoleic acid. Omega-3, or linolenic acid, on the other hand, is relatively difficult to obtain in the usual food choices. Among plant sources only soybeans and the oil from rapeseed (canola oil), black walnut, linseed and flaxseed have appreciable amounts of omega-3. Wild plants and herbs *do* contain substantial amounts of linolenic acid, however … but domesticated grasses and grains contain almost none. And it follows, therefore, that the meat from animals raised on domesticated grasses and grains also contains very low levels of linolenic acid.

Linoleic acid and linolenic acid have no direct role in human metabolism … rather they are the starting point of very critical, yet different metabolic pathways. Linoleic acid, or omega-6, initiates a pathway leading to arachidonic acid, which in turn is the beginning point for pathways to a large number of specific bio-chemical reactions and functions. One critical series of such pathways lead to inflammatory and coagulation responses in various parts of the body which are essential to immunization and repair functions.

Linolenic acid, or omega-3, on-the-other-hand, initiates a pathway in a very different, almost antagonistic direction, leading to docosahexaenoic acid (DHA) and eicosapentaenoic acid (EPA). DHA and EPA are then the beginning point for a series of reactions and metabolic pathways leading, for example, to anti-inflammatory and anti-coagulation responses. DHA and EPA are thus considered to be nutrition factors in preventing inflammation in joints and various parts of the body, and in preventing the formation of arterial plague, or atherosclerosis.

It is difficult to obtain sufficient linolenic acid, or omega-3, in our usual American diet, except, that is, for one source, which is actually a short-cut … and that is by obtaining pre-formed DHA and EPA from fish, and especially the oil of so-called 'fatty fish', such as salmon and cod.

Our knowledge and interest in linoleic and linolenic acid was largely prompted by studies of Greenland Eskimos in the 1970's. This population consumed a diet consisting almost entirely of fish … but heart disease and atherosclerosis was almost non-existent among the Greenland Eskimos. The high amount of DHA and EPA in their diet protected them from excessive inflammation and coagulation. However, a simple nose bleed could kill them.

These two separate pathways, one beginning with omega-6, and the other with omega-3, are *not* regulated by any automatic or homeostatic function. The question *why* is one of the mysteries of our physiology and our physical evolution. One theory is that our ancestors, at some time in our early humanoid development, likely lived in an environment so rich with both omega-6 and omega-3 that there was no need for a homeostatic function to regulate the separate pathways and, in particular, to determine which pathway should have priority under any given set of circumstances.

This predicament is further complicated by the fact that both pathways are very slow, and are vulnerable to disruption by factors such as the presence of strong anti-oxidants… this is especially true with the omega-3 pathway. DHA and EPA, for example, are easily destroyed by heat, and it has been reported that a daily intake of as little as 200 mg of the anti-oxidant vitamin E is sufficient to obstruct the pathway from linolenic acid to DHA and EPA.

The determination of the relative influence of either pathway over the other then depends solely on the amounts consumed and successfully digested, within a given time period. The ratio of the intake amounts then becomes critical. Our National Academy of Sciences currently recommends a ratio of 13:1, in favor of omega-6.

I will return to this discussion in the next chapter ... and I delve into this topic much deeper in other parts of *The Nutrition Factor: A Bold New Perspective*.

However ... how does this all relate to cow's milk? Well, it just so happens that a single glass of whole milk contains an average of 1.35 grams of omega-3, or 12.6% of our recommended daily intake. Four glasses would then provide over 50% of our requirement. The relative amount of omega-6 in cow's milk is less, but this could be considered a blessing considering that omega-6 is more readily available in other foods, and the danger of overwhelming the omega-3 is thus diminished.

The relative availability of linolenic acid, or omega-3, in cow's milk, compared with linoleic acid, or omega-6, has been theorized to be a possible factor in the reported lowered risk of chronic disease and lowered blood pressure associated with the consumption of milk.

Milk fat and cardiovascular disease

There has been a great deal written on the subject of saturated fat and its association with cardiovascular disease, most notably the build-up of plaque in the arteries, or atherosclerosis. This association was what prompted the great shift from milk butter to vegetable oils in the 1950s. Since that time numerous additional studies have supported this relationship. However, the controversy is not fully resolved. For one thing, we now know that 'saturated fat' is not 'saturated fat', meaning that there are several fatty acids contained under the general classification of 'saturated fat', and they do not all have the same atherosclerotic effect.

One recent study suggests that the impact of dairy foods and milk fat on cardiovascular disease risk is over-estimated. German et al, in his study entitled *A reappraisal of the impact of dairy foods and milk fat on cardiovascular disease risk,* concludes: "Despite the contribution of dairy products to the saturated fatty acid composition of the diet, and given the diversity of dairy foods of widely differing composition, there is no clear evidence that dairy food consumption is consistently associated with a higher risk of CVD." (German, 2009)

A note about Mad Cow Disease

The scientific name for 'Mad Cow Disease' is *bovine spongiform encephalitis* (BSE), and is a disease that affects the nervous system and is caused by an infectious protein called a *prion*. The disease can be transmitted to humans via consumption of meat from infected cattle. In humans the disease is known as *transmissible spongiform encephalopathy* or *variant Creutzfeidt-Jacob disease*. However, to date the infectious prion protein has not been found in bovine milk ... you cannot get Mad Cow's Disease by drinking cow's milk.

Designer milk

With increased knowledge and more sophisticated technology, it is entirely within our present-day capabilities to improve the nutritional benefits of cow's milk. Altering a dairy cow's feed and environment can potentially pass on enhanced nutrient compositions in milk. New technologies now enable us to modify milk properties and create increased benefit.

One study has identified a previously overlooked form of calcium within the casein proteins, called 'micellar calcium phosphate' (MCP) which is much more bioavailable than the normal calcium carbonate. The higher bioavailability is thought to be due to the greater solubility of the MCP-CPP complex in the small intestine. The authors, Aoki and Aoe, suggest that this more bioavailable form of milk protein could assist in the prevention of osteoporosis. (Aoki, T.; Aoe, S.; *Prevention of osteoporosis by foods and supplements. Bioavailability of milk micellar calcium phosphate, 2006)*

Another study by Itabashi (2006) concludes that "milk whey protein, especially its basic protein fraction (milk basic protein: MBP), contains components capable of promoting bone formation and inhibiting bone resorption." This researcher concludes that "MBP supplementation could be effective for bone health in a wide range of the population, especially those who hate to drink milk."

Possible associations with reduced risk for chronic diseases and weight control

Over the years a large number of research studies, literature reviews, and expert comment have been directed to the perceived general 'good' of cow's milk and other dairy products, and the possible association with a decrease in the risk for various chronic diseases, for lowering blood pressure, and for weight control and the prevention of obesity. In this section I have listed a number of these articles, with their authors, article title and topic, citation information, *and* conclusions. The source for these articles include PubMed (NIH), library research in periodicals and books, and books from my own collection. I have compiled a similar list at the end of Chapter Three, The 'Bad'. Almost all of these articles are easy to access online, particularly the PubMed articles, although full texts usually must be purchased.

Additional references ... with conclusions and comments ... for Chapter Two

The following references do not encompass the total of all the studies competed in this field. They are, however, most of what surfaced through a PubMed and library search. In addition, I have omitted articles that are statements only or are purely 'expert opinion' ... we have more than enough of that floating around !!

Bone growth and maintenance, and osteoporosis

Berkey, C.S.; Colditz, G.A.; Rockett, H.R.; Frazier, A.L.; Willett, W.C.; *Dairy consumption and female height growth: prospective cohort study.* Cancer Epidemiology And Prevention, 2009, June, 18(6): 1881-7. A cohort prospective study of 5,101 U.S. girls. Conclusion: "Of the foods/nutrients studied, dairy protein had the strongest association with height growth. These findings suggest that a factor in the nonlipid phase of milk, but not protein itself, has growth-promoting action in girls."

Bonjour, J.P.; Brandolini-Bunion, M.; Boirie, Y.; Morel-Laporte, F.; Braesco, V.; Bertiere, M.C.; Souberbielle, J.C.; *Inhibition of bone turnover by milk intake in postmenopausal women,* British Journal of Nutrition, 2008, October; 100(4): 866-74. Prospective cross-over study of 30 postmenopausal women. Conclusion: "In conclusion, a 6-week period of milk supplementation induced a decrease in several biochemical variables compatible with diminished bone turnover mediated by reduction in parathyroid hormone secretion. This nutritional approach to postmenopausal alteration in bone metabolism may be a valuable measure in the primary prevention of osteoporosis."

Chang, S.C.; O'Brien, K.O.; Nathanson, M.S.; Caulfield, L.E.; Mancini, J.; Witter, F.R.; *Fetal femur length is influenced by maternal dairy intake in pregnant African American adolescents.* A retrospective chart review of 1120 pregnant African American adolescents. Conclusion: "... consumption of less than 2 servings of dairy products/day by pregnant adolescents may negatively affect fetal bone development by limiting the amount of calcium provided to the fetus."

Esterie, L.; Sabatier, S.B.; Guiilon-Metz, P.; Walrant-Debray, O.; Guaydier-Souquieres, G.; Jehan, F.; Garabedian, M.; *Milk, rather than other foods, is associated with vertebral bone mass and circulating IGF-1 in female adolescents.* Osteoporosis International, 2009, April; 20(4): 567-75. Clinical study of 193 healthy adolescent girls. Conclusion: "Girls with milk intakes below 55 mL/day have significantly lower BMD (bone mineral density), BMC (bone mineral content), and IGF-1 and higher PTH (hormones) compared to girls consuming over 260 mL/day. ... Milk consumption, preferably to other calcium sources, is associated with lumbar BMC and BMD in postmenarcheal girls."

Florito, L.M.; Mitchell, D.C.; Smiciklas-Wright, H.; Birch, L.L.; *Girls' calcium intake is associated with bone mineral content during middle childhood.* Journal of Nutrition, 2006, May, 136(5(: 1281-6. A 6-year time study of 151 non-Hispanic white girls. Conclusion: "Results from the present study provide new longitudinal evidence that calcium intake, especially calcium from dairy foods, can have a favorable effect on girls' TBBMC during middle childhood."

Huncharek, M.; Muscat, J.; Kupeinick, B.; *Impact of dairy products and dietary calcium on bone-mineral content in children: results of a meta-analysis.* A review and meta-analysis of 21 randomized controlled trials. Conclusion: "Increased dietary calcium/dairy products, with and without vitamin D, significantly increases total body and lumber spine BMC in children with low base-line intakes."

Nieves, J.W.; Barrett-Connor, E.; Siris, E.S.; Zion, M.; Barlas, S.; Chen, Y.T.; *Calcium and vitamin D intake influence bone mass, but not short-term fracture risk, in Caucasian postmenopausal women from the National Osteoporosis Risk Assessment (NORA) study,* Osteoporosis International, 2008, May; 19(5): 673-9. An observation and statistical analysis study of 76,507 postmenopausal women at baseline and after 3 years. Conclusion: "Thus, higher calcium and vitamin D intakes significantly reduced the odds of osteoporosis but not the 3-year risk of fracture in these Caucasian women."

North American Menopause Society; *The role of calcium in peri- and postmenopausal women: 2006 position statement of the North American Menopause Society,* Menopause, 2006, Nov-Dec; 13(6): 878-80. Statement: "Adequate calcium intake (in the presence of adequate vitamin D status) has been shown to reduce bone loss in peri- and postmenopausal women and reduce fractures in postmenopausal women older than age 60 with low calcium intakes. Adequate calcium is considered a key component of any bone-protective therapeutic regimen. Calcium has also been associated with beneficial effects in several non-skeletal disorders, primarily hypertension, colorectal cancer, obesity, and nephrolithiasis, although the extent of those effects has not been fully elucidated. The calcium requirement rises at menopause. The largest calcium intake for most postmenopausal women in 1,200 mg/day. Adequate vitamin D status, defined as 30 ng/mL or more of serum 25-hydroxyvitamin D (usually achieved with a daily oral intake of at least 400 to 600 IU), is required to achieve the nutritional benefits of calcium. The best source of calcium is food, and the best food source is dairy products."

Calcium

Buzinaro, E.F.; Almeida, R.N.; Mazelo, G.M.; *Bioavailability of dietary calcium,* Arquivos Brasilieros de Endocrinologia & Metabologia, 2006, October; 50(5): 852-61. Clinical and lab studies. Conslusion: "The richest and best-absorbed calcium source is cow's milk and its derivatives."

Hearney, R.P.; *Calcium intake and disease prevention,* Arquivos Brasileiros de Endocrinologia & Metabologia, 2006, Aug; 50(4): 685-93. A review of previous studies. Conclusion:"Adequate calcium intakes (1000-1500 mg/d) in adults have been shown in controlled trials to lower the risk of osteoprotic factures, kidney stones, obesity, and hypertension. The best source of calcium is dairy foods, largely because the disorders concerned depend upon multiple nutrients, not just calcium, and dairy provides a broad array of essential nutrients in addition to calcium, and at low cost.

Cancer

Alvarez-Leon, E.E.; Roman-Vinas, B.; Serra-Majem, L.; *Dairy products and health: a review of the epidemiological evidence.* A review of epidemiological evidence. Conclusion: "There is no evidence of an association between the consumption of dairy products and breast cancer."

Holt, P.R.; Wolper, C.; Moss, S.F.; Yang, K.; Lipkin, M.; *Comparison of calcium supplementation or low-fat dairy foods on epithelial cell proliferation and differentiation.* Nutrition And Cancer, 2001, 41(1-2): 150-5. An observational cross-over 'head-to-head' study of 40 subjects at risk for colonic neoplasia. Conclusion: "These data indicate that increased dietary calcium given as supplements in the diet or in the diet in low-fat dairy foods lowers epithelial cell proliferation indexes from a higher-to-a-lower-risk pattern."

Huncharek, M.; Muscat, J.; Kupelnick, B.; *Dairy products, dietary calcium and vitamin D intake as risk factors for prostate cancer: a meta-analysis of 26,769 cases from 45 observational studies.* Nutrition And Cancer, 2008, 60(4): 421-41. A meta-analysis study. Conclusion: "The data from observational studies do not support an association between dairy product use and an increased risk of prostate cancer."

Moorman, P.G.; Terry, P.D.; *Consumption of dairy products and the risk of breast cancer: a review of the literature,* American Journal of Clinical Nutrition, 2004, July; 80(1): 5-14. A review of previous studies. Conclusion: "The available epidemiologic evidence does not support a strong association between the consumption of milk or other dairy products and breast cancer risk."

Pufulete, M.; *Intake of dairy products and risk of colorectal neoplasia,* Nutrition Research Reviews, 2008, June; 21(1): 56-67. A review of previous prospective cohort studies. Conclusion: "Prospective cohort studies suggest that higher intakes of dairy products, in particular milk, are associated with a decreased risk of colorectal cancer (CRC)."

Koralek, D.O.; Bertone-Johnson, E.R.; Leitzmann, M.F.; Sturgeon, S.R.; Lacey, J.V. Jr.; Schairer, C.; Schatzkin, A.; *Relationship between calcium, lactose, vitamin D, and dairy products and ovarian cancer.* A review of two prospective studies. Nutrition and Cancer, 2006, September; Vol. 56, Issue 1: 22-30 Conclusion: "No statistically significant relations were found for consumption of specific dairy foods, lactose, or vitamin D and ovarian cancer risk."

Parodi, R.W.; *A role for milk proteins and their peptides in cancer prevention,* Current Pharmaceutical Design, 2007; 13(8): 813-28. A review of animal studies. Conclusion: "...animal studies suggest that certain peptides and amino acids derived from dietay proteins may influence carcinogenesis. The predominant protein in milk, casein, its peptides, but not liberated amino acids, have antimutagenic properties. Animal models, usually for colon and mammary tumorgenesis, nearly always show that whey protein is superior to other dietary proteins for suppression of tumour development."

Tsuda, H.; Sekine, K.; *Milk Components as Cancer Chemopreventive Agents,* Asian Pacific Journal of Cancer Prevention, 2000; 1(4): 277-282. A review of epidemiological studies. Conclusion: "It has been proposed that whereas fats in general might promote tumor development, individual milk fats like conjugated linoleic acid and glycosh/lingolipids could exert inhibitory effects. There is also considerable evidence that calcium in milk products protects against colon cancer, while promoting in the prostate through suppression of circulating levels of 1,25 dihydroxyvitamin D. Whey protein may also be beneficial, as shown by both animal and human studies, and experimental data have demonstrated that the major component bovine lactoferrin (bLF), inhibits colon carcinogenesis in the post-initiation stage in male F344 rats treated with azoxymethane (AOM) without any overt toxicity. Results in other animal models have provided further indications that bovine lactoferrin might find application as a natural ingredient of milk with potential for chemoprevention of colon and other cancers."

Cardiovascular disease

Gibson, R.A.; Makrides, M.; Smithers, L.G.; Voevodin, M.; Sinclair, A.J.; *The effect of dairy foods on CHD: a systematic review of prospective cohort studies,* British Journal of Nutrition, 2009, November; 102(9): 1267-75. A review of 12 prospective cohort studies involving more than 280,000 subjects. Conclusion: "Although dairy foods contribute to the SFA (saturated fatty acid) composition of the diet, this systematic review could find no consistent evidence that dairy food consumption is associated with a higher risk of CHD."

Kontogianni, M.D.; Panagiotakos, D.B.; Pitsavos, C.; Stefanadis, C.; *Modelling dairy intake on the development of acute coronary syndromes: the CARDIO2000 study,* European Journal of Cardiovascular Prevention & Rehabilitation, 2006, October: 13(5); 791-

7. A cross-sectional controlled observation study of 700 males and 148 females with first event of an acute coronary syndrome and 1078 population based controls. Conclusion: "Dairy consumption seems to offer significant protection against coronary heart disease, irrespective of various clinical, lifestyle and other characteristics of the participants."

McGill, C.R.; Fulgoni, V.L. 3rd; DiRienzo, D.; Huth, P.J.; Kurlich, A.C.; Miller, G.D.; *Contribution of dairy products to dietary potassium intake in the United States population,* Journal of the American College of Nutrition, 2008, February, 27(1): 44-50. Meta-analysis of NHANES survey data 1999-2002. Conclusion: "Adequate dietary potassium is associated with a reduced risk of cardiovascular and other chronic diseases ... Mean and median potassium intakes increased with increasing dairy intake but were below current intake recommendations for all age groups analyzed."

Pins, J.J.; Keenan, J.M.; *Effects of whey peptides on cardiovascular disease risk factors,* Journal of Clinical Hypertension, 2006, November; 8(11): 775-82. A controlled study of 30 prehypertensive subjects. Conclusion: "Whey-derived peptides might be a viable treatment option for prehypertensive and/or stage 1 hypertensive populations."

Tholstrup, T.; *Dairy products and cardiovascular disease.* Current Opinion in Lipidology, 2006, February, 17(1): 1-10. A review. Conclusion: "There is no strong evidence that dairy products increase the risk of coronary heart disease in healthy men of all ages or young and middle-aged healthy women.

Chronic diseases

Azadbakht, L.; Mirmiran, P.; Esmailzadeh, A.; Azizi, F.; *Dairy consumption is inversely associated with the prevalence of the metabolic syndrome in Tehranian adults,* American Journal of Clinical Nutrition, 2005, September; 82(3): 523-30. A cross-sectional study of 357 men and 470 women. Conclusion: "Dairy consumption is inversely associated with the risk of having metabolic syndrome."

Suhara, W.; Koide, H.; Okuzawa, T.; Hayashi, D.; Hashimoto, T.; Kojo, .; *Cow's milk increases the activities of human nuclear receptors peroxisome proliferator-activated receptors alpha and delta and retinoid X receptor alpha involved in the regulation of energy homeostasis, obesity, and inflammation.* Journal of Dairy Science, 2009, September, 92(9): 4180-7. Laboratory test results. Conclusion: "This study unambiguously clarified at the celluar level that cow's milk increased the activities of human PPARalpha, PPARdelta, and RXRalpha ... PPAR agonists have the potential to prevent or ameliorate diseases such as hyperlipidemia, diabetes, atherosclerosis, and obesity."

Dental caries

Merritt, J.; Qi, F.; Shi, W.; *Milk helps build strong teeth and promotes oral health.* Journal of the California Dental Association, 2006, May, 34(5): 361-6. A review. Conclusion: "A great deal of research into the benefits of milk consumption has gone largely under the radar for many decades. There is a wealth of studies both in the United States and abroad to suggest that milk consumption is largely anti-cariogenic when combined with a typical routine of oral hygiene."

Simazaki, Y.; Shirota, T.; Uchida, K.; Yonemoto, K.; Kiyohara, Y.; Iida, M.; Saito, T.; Yamashita, Y.; *Intake of dairy products and periodontal diesese: the Hisayama Study,* Journal of Periodontology, 2008, January; 79(1): 131-7. Clinical study of 942 residents aged 40 to 79 years in Hisayama Town, Fukuoka, Japan. Conclusion: "...the subjects eating 55 grams or more of lactic acid foods (dairy foods) had a significantly lower prevalence of deep PD (probing depth) and severe CAL (clinical attachment loss) compared to those not eating these foods."

Diabetes

Choi, H.K.; Willett, W.C.; Stampfer, M.J.; Rimm, E.; Hu, F.B.; *Dairy consumption and risk of type 2 diabetes mellitus in men: a prospective study,* Archives of Internal Medicine, 2005, May 9; 165(9): 997-1003. A prospective study of 41,254 male participants with no history of diabetes, cardiovascular disease, and cancer at baseline, followed-up for 12 years ... the Health Professionals Follow-up Study. Conclusions: "Dietary patterns characterized by higher dairy intake, especially low-fat dairy intake, may lower the risk of type 2 diabetes in men."

Liu, S.; Choi, H.K.; Ford, E.; Song, Y.; Klevak, A.; Buring, J.E.; Manson, J.E.; *A prospective study of dairy intake and the risk of type 2 diabetes in women,* Diabetes Care, 2006, July; 29(7): 1579-84. A 10-year follow-up study of 37,183 women. Conclusion: "A dietary pattern that incorporates higher low-fat dairy products may lower the risk of type 2 diabetes in middle-aged or older women."

Pfeuffer, M.; Schrezenmyer J; *Milk and the metabolic syndrome,* Obesity Reviews, 2007, March; 8(2): 109-18. Review of previous studies. Conclusion: "The metabolic syndrome is a cluster of metabolic disorders, namely dyslipdaemia, obesity and glucose intolerance. Insulin resistance is the core phenomenon. In several studies dairy consumption was inversely associated with the occurrence of one or several facets of the metabolic syndrome."

Tremblay, A.; Gilbert, J.A.; *Milk products, insulin resistance syndrome and type 2 diabetes.* Journal of the American College of Nutrition, 2009, February; 28 Suppl 1: 91S-102S. A review of various studies. Conclusion: "Overall, the intake of low-fat dairy products is a feature of a healthy dietary pattern which has been shown to contribute to a significant extent to the prevention of IRS (insulin resistance syndrome)."

Jaffiol, C.; *Milk and dairy products in the prevention and therapy of obesity, type 2 diabetes and metabolic syndrome,* Bulletin del Academie Nationale de Medecine (Paris), 2008, April; 192(4): 749-58. A review of prospective trials. Conclusion: "Milk and dairy foods are recommended for patients with obesity, diabetes, hypertension and metabolic syndrome, and also for patients at risk."

Martini, L.A.; Wood, R.J.; *Milk intake and the risk of type 2 diabetes mellitus, hypertension and prostate cancer,* Arquivos Brasileiros de Endocrinologia and Metabologia, 2009, July; 53(5): 688-94. Analysis of previous studies. Conclusion: "Based on the current evidence, it is possible that milk/dairy products, when consumed in adequate amounts and mainly with reduced fat content, has beneficial effect on the prevention of hyptertension and diabetes."

Hypertension

Wang, L.; Manson, J.E.; Buring, J.E.; Lee, I.M.; Sesso, H.D.; *Dietary intake of dairy products, calcium, and vitamin D and the risk of hypertension in middle-aged and older women,* Hypertension, 2008, April, 51(4): 1073-9. Epub 2008 Feb 7. A prospective cohort study, 28,886 U.S. women were followed up over 10 years. Conclusion: "Our study found that intakes of low-fat dairy products, calcium, and vitamin D were each inversely associated with risk of hypertension in middle-aged and older women, suggesting their potential roles in the primary prevention of hypertension and cardiovascular complications."

Djousse', L.; Pankow, J.S.; Hunt, S.C.; Heiss, G.; Province, M.A.; Kabagambe, E.K.; Ellison, R.C.; *Influence of saturated fat and linolenic acid on the association between intake of dairy products and blood pressure.* American Journal of Epidemiology, 1996; 143: 1219-28 An analysis of data from the National Heart, Lung, and Blood Institute Family Heart Study, 4,797 participants. Conclusion: "Our data indicate an inverse association between dairy consumption and prevalent hypertension (HTN) that was independent of dietary calcium."

Ruidavets, J.B.; Bongard, V.; Simon, C.; Dallongeville, J.; Ducimetiere, P.' Arveiler, D.; Amouyel, P.; Bingham, A.; Ferrieres, J.; *Independent contribution of dairy products and calcium intake to blood pressure variations at a population level.* Journal of Hypertension, 2006, April, 24(4): 671-8. A randomized cross-sectional study of 912 men aged 45-64. Conclusion: "Dairy products and dietary calcium are both significantly and independently associated with low levels of systolic blood pressure."

Toledo, E.; Delgado-Rodriguez, M.; Estruch, R.; Salas-Salvado, J.; Corella, D.; Gomez-Gracia, E.; Fiol, M.; Lamuela-Raventos, R.M.; Schroder, H.; Aros, F.; Rulz-Gutierrez, V.; Lapetra, J.; Conde-Herrera, M. Saez, G.; Vinyoles, E.; Marinez-Gonzales, M.A; *Low-fat dairy products and blood pressure: follow-up of 2290 older persons at high cardiovascular risk participating in the PREDIMED study,* British Journal of Nutrition, 2009, January; 101(1): 59-57. Conclusion: "Intake of low-fat dairy products was inversely associated with BP (blood pressure) in an older population at high cardiovascular risk."

Wang, L.; Manson, J.E.; Buring, J.E.; Lee, I.M.; Sesso, H.D.; *Dietary intake of dairy products, calcium, and vitamin D and the risk of hypertension in middle-aged and older women,* Hypertension, 2008, April; 51(4): 1073-9. A prospective cohort study of 28,886 U.S. women. Conclusion: "Our study found that intakes of low-fat dairy products, calcium, and vitamin D were each inversely associated with risk of hypertension in middle-aged and older women."

Xu, J.Y.; Qin, L.G.; Wang, P.Y.; Li, W.; Chang, C.: *Effect of milk tripeptides on blood pressure: a meta-analysis of randomized controlled trials,* Nutrition, 2008, October; 24(10): 933-40. An analysis of 12 previous studies. Conclusion: "Our analysis provided evidence that milk-derived tripeptides have hypotensive effects in prehypertensive and hypertensive subjects."

Lactose intolerance

BBC NEWS; *China drinks its milk,* BBC News, Tuesday, 7 August, 2007. Statements: "China's growing love of dairy products is threatening to push UK prices up. But why are the Chinese drinking more milk and why does it affect the whole world ... Wen Jiabao, Chinese Premier: 'I have a dream to provide every Chinese, especially children, sufficient milk each day' ... The one confusing factor is that of lactose intolerance. The majority of Chinese adults suffer a deficiency of lactase, the enzyme needed to break down the lactose in milk and the common trigger for lactose intolerance. ... Cheese and processed milk products are low in lactose (in China), there is lactose-free milk, and there are many adults that suffer no, or only limited, intolerance."

Brannon, P.M.; Carpenter, T.O.; Fernandez, J.R.; Gilsanz, V.; Gould, J.B.; Hall, K.E.; Hui S.L.; Lupton, J.R.; Mennela, J.; Miller, N.J.; Osganian, S.K.; Sellmeyer, D.E.; Suchy, F.J.; Wolf, M.A.*; NIH Consensus Development Conference Statement: Lactose Intolerance and Health*, National Institute of Health (NIH) Consensus Statement, Science Statements, 2010, February 24;27(2) Conclusions: "(1) Lactose intolerance is a real and important clinical syndrome, but its true prevalence is not known. (2) The majority of people with lactose malabsorption do not have clinical lactose intolerance. Many individuals who think they are lactose intolerant are not lactose malabsorbers. (3) Many individuals with real or perceived lactose intolerance avoid dairy and inadequate amounts of calcium and vitamin D which may predispose them to decreased bone accrual, osteoporosis, and other adverse health outcomes. In most cases, individuals do not need to eliminate dairy consumption completely." www.ncbi.nlm.nih.gov/pubmed/20186234

Fuller, F.; Beghin, J.C.; *China's Growing Market for Dairy Products,*CARD,www.card.iastate.edu/iowa_ag_review/summer_04/article5.aspx Statements: (1) China has one of the lowest levels of per capita milk consumption in the world, averaging just about 5.6 kilograms per person per year (2003). While rural consumption has grown little, urban consumption has increased 25 percent 1997 – 2002. (2) Contrary to popular belief, dairy products have a long history in China.

Gaskin, D.J.; Llich, J.Z.; *Lactose Maldigestion Revisited: Diagnosis, Prevalence in Ethnic Minorities, and Dietary Recommendations to Overcome It,* American Journal of Lifestyle Medicine, Vol. 3, Number 3; 212-18, 2009. A review article. Conclusion: "Clinical trials show that even those individuals who do maldigest lactose could overcome adverse symptoms by a few simple dietary strategies. In addition, new research points to possible manipulation toward alleviating symptoms."

Hovde; Farup, P.G.; *A comparison of diagnostic tests for lactose malabsorption – which one is best?,* BMC Gastroenterology, 2009, October 31; 9:82 Conclusion: "A lactose breath test with measurement of H2 +CH4x2 in expired air had the best diagnostic properties.

Jarvis, J.K.; Miller, G.D.; *Overcoming the barrier of lactose intolerance to reduce health disparities.* Journal of the National Medical Association, 2002, February; 94(2): 55-66. Statement by the National Dairy Council. Conclusion: "The high incidence figures for primary lactose maldigesion among minority groups grossly overestimates the number who will experience intolerance symptoms after drinking a glass of milk with a meal."

Johnson, A.O.; Semenya, J.G.; Buchowski, M.S.; Enwonwu, C.O.; Scrimshaw, N.S.; *Correlation of lactose maldigestion, lactose intolerance, and milk intolerance.* American Journal of Clinical Nutrition, 1993, 57: 399-401. Clinical test of 164 African Americans aged 12 to 40 years who claimed intolerance to one cup of milk. Conclusion: "The results suggest that the cause of milk intolerance in as many as one-third of African Americans claiming symptoms after ingestion of a moderate amount of milk cannot be its lactose content."

Johnson, A.O.; Semenya, J.G.; Buchowski, M.S.; Enwonwu, C.O.; Scrimshaw, N.S.; *Adaptation of lactose maldigesters to continued milk intakes,* American Journal of Clinical Nutrition, 1993, 58: 879-81. Clinical tests of 25 lactose-maldigesting and lactose intolerant African Americans, 13 to 39 years of age. Conclusion: "This study suggests that the majority of African-American young adults who claim intolerance to moderate amounts of milk can ultimately adapt and tolerate greater-than-or-equal-to the grams of lactose in milk equivalent to 8 oz. of full-lactose milk with minimal or no discomfort if milk is ingested in gradually increasing amounts. The mechanism of adaptation is assumed to be an increased tolerance to colonic lactose-fermentation products."

Moore, B.J.; *Dairy Foods: Are They Politically Correct?,* Nutrition Today, 2003, May-June; 38(3): 82-90. A review of the evidence on the prevalence and management of verified lactose intolerance. Conclusion: "The genetically programmed ability to digest the milk sugar lactose normally declines throughout childhood in all ethnic groups. Only rarely does lactase nonpersitence result in verifiable lactose intolerance. The intolerance-gastrointestinal symptoms, such as diarrhea, bloating, and abdominal cramping is easily managed when it occurs and is not a barrier to the consumption of 2 to 3 servings of calcium-rich dairy foods, as encouraged by the Dietary Guideline for Americans."

National Medical Association; *Lactose intolerance and African Americans: implications for the consumption of appropriate intake levels of key nutrients,* Journal of the National Medical Association, 2009, October; 101(10 Suppl): 5S-23S. Statement conclusion: "Since dairy nutrients address important health concerns, the amelioration of lactose intolerance is an investment in health. Lactose intolerance is common, is easy to treat, and can be managed. It is possible to consume dairy even in the face of a history of maldigestion or lactose intolerant issues. Gradually increasing lactose in the diet – drinking small milk portions with food, eating yogurt, and consuming cheese – are effective strategies for managing lactose intolerance and meeting optimal dairy needs."

O'Connell, S.; Walsh, G.; *A novel acid-stable, acid-active beta-galactosidase potentially suited to the alleviation of lactose intolerance,* Applied Microbiology and Biotechnology, 2010, March; 86(2): 517-24. A clinical analysis study. Conclusion: "The acid-stable, acid-active enzyme, along with the novel two-segment delivery system, may prove beneficial in the more effective treatment of lactose intolerance."

Scrimshaw, N.S.; Murray, E.; *Lactose tolerance and milk consumption: myths and realities,* Archivos Latinoamericanos de Nutricion, 1988; September; 38(3): 543-67. This is an early study and expert opinion much referenced, and used as a reference for WHO's position on lactose intolerance worldwide. Dr. Nevin Scrimshaw is a world renowned nutritionist and a true 'giant' in the field. Conclusion: "Prevalence of lactose non-digestors in Latin American populations ranges from 45% to 100%. However, this is not a reliable predictor of the acceptability of milk and milk products containing lactose. Milk is being used successfully for the supplementary feeding of children worldwide, and most lactose non-digesters' can tolerate at least 240 ml of milk or the lactose equivalent in other products. Lactose maldigestion does not interfere with the absorption of the protein and essential micronutrients in milk."

Political correctness

Moore, B.J.; *Dairy Foods: Are They Politically Correct?*, Nutrition Today, 2003, May-June; 28(3): 82-90. Conclusion: "This article considers the scientific evidence on the prevalence and management of verified lactose intolerance and the growing misperception that dairy foods should be avoided because ethnic populations cannot tolerate them ... The intolerance-gastrointestinal symptoms, such as diarrhea, bloating, and abdominal cramping is easily managed when it occurs and is not a barrier to the consumption of 2 to 3 servings of calcium-rich dairy foods, as encouraged by the Dietary Guideline for Americans."

Psoriasis

Drouin, R.; Lamiot, E.; Cantin, K.; Gauthier, S.F.; Pouliot, Y.; Poubelle, P.E.; Juneau, C.; *XP=828L (Dermylex), a new whey protein extract with potential benefit for mild to moderate psoriasis,* Canadian Journal of Physiology and Pharmacology, 2007, September: 85(9): 943-51. Results of clinical trials. Conclusion: "XP-828L, a whey protein extract, has demonstrated potential benefits or the treatment of mild to moderate psoriasis."

Stroke

Elwood, P.C.; Strain, J.J.; Robson, P.J.; Fehily, A.M.; Hughes, J.; Pickering, J.; Ness, A.; *Milk consumption, stroke, and heart attack risk: evidence from the Caerphilly cohort of older men,* Journal of Epedemiology & Community Health,2005, June; 59(6): 502-6. A 20 year follow-up study of 665 men in South Wales. Conclusion: "...the subjects who drank more than the median amount of milk had a reduced risk of ischaemic stroke."

Massey, L.K.; *Dairy food consumption, blood pressure and stroke,* Journal of Nutrition, 2001, July, 131(7):1875-8. A review of two prospective studies. Conclusion: "The two prospective studies of dairy food consumption and stroke incidence both indicate that a higher intake of dairy foods reduces risk."

Weight control, obesity

Carruth, B.R.; Skinner, J.D.; *The role of dietary calcium and other nutrients in moderating body fat in preschool children.* International Journal of Obesity (London), 2005, April, 29(4): 388-90. A longitudinal study of 53 children over 2-96 months. Conclusion: Higher longitudinal intakes of calcium, monounsaturated fat, and servings of dairy products were associated with lower body fat."

Eagan, M.S.; Lyle, R.M.; Bunther, C.W.; Peacock, M.; Teegarden, D.; *Effect of 1-year dairy product intervention on fat mass in young women: 6-month follow-up,* Obesity (Silver Spring), 2008, December; 14(2): 2242-8. A randomized study of 154 young women. Conclusion: "Dietary calcium intake over 18 months predicted a negative change in body fat mass. Thus, increased dietary calcium intakes through dairy products may prevent fat mass accumulation in young, healthy, normal-weight women."

Ebringer, L.; Ferenci, M.; Krajcovic, J.; *Beneficial health effects of milk and fermented dairy products – review,* Folia Microbiologica, 2008; 53(5): 378-94. A review of previous studies. Conclusion: "There has been growing evidence of the role that dairy proteins play in the regulation of satiety, food intake and obesity-related metabolic disorders."

Heaney, R.P.; Davies, K.M.; Barger-Lux, M.J.; *Calcium and weight: clinical studies.* Journal of the American College of Nurition, 2002, April, 21(2): 152S-155S. Re-analysis of 6 observational studies and 3 controlled trials in which calcium intake was the independent variable. Conclusion: "Taken together these data suggest that increasing calcium intake by the equivalent of two dairy servings per day could reduce the risk of overweight substantially, perhaps by as much as 70 percent.

Major, G.C.; Chaput, J.P.; Ledoux, M.; St-Pierre, S.; Anderson, G.H.; Zemel M.B.; Tremblay, A.; *Recent developments in calcium-related obesity research.* Obesity Reviews, 2008, September, 9(5): 428-45. Review of discussion by subject experts during a symposium. Conclusion: "...calcium and dairy food intake can influence many components of energy and fat balance, indicating that inadequate calcium/dairy intake may increase the risk of positive energy imbalance and of other health problems."

Moore, L.L.; Bradlee, M.L.; Gao, D.; Singer, M.R.; *Low dairy intake in early childhood predicts excess body fat gain.* Obesity, 2006, June, 14(6): 1010-8. A longitudinal follow-through study of the children of the original 106 families enrolled in the Framington Children's Study, aged from 5 to 13 years of age. Conclusion: "Suboptimal dairy intakes during preschool in this cohort were associated with greater gains in body fat throughout childhood."

46

Novotny, R.; Daida, Y.G.; Acharya, S.; Grove, J.S.; Vogt, T.M.; *Dairy intake is associated with lower body fat and soda intake with greater weight in adolescent girls.* Journal of Nutrition, 2004, August, 134(8): 1905-9. Clinical study of 323 9-14 year old girls in Hawaii. Conclusion: "Dairy intake is associated with lower body fat and soda intake with greater weight in adolescent girls."

Palacios, C.; Benedetti, P.; Fonseca, S.; *Impact of calcium intake on body mass index in Venezuelan adolescents.* Puerto Rico Health Sciences Journal, 2007, September; 26(3): 199-204. Clinical study of 100 adolescents. Conclusion: "... we found that high calcium intake in young boys was related to a lower BMI (body mass index)."

Shahar, D.R.; Abel, R.; Elhayany, A.; Vardi, H.; Fraser, D.; *Does dairy calcium intake enhance weight toss among overweight diabetic patients?* Diabetes Care, 2007, March, 30(3): 485-9. A randomized clinical trial of 259 diabetic patients. Conclusion: "A diet rich in dairy calcium intake enhances weight reduction in type 2 diabetic patients."

Teegarden, D.; *Calcium intake and reduction in weight or fat mass,* Journal of Nutrition, 2003, January; 133(1): 249S-251S. A review of clinical trials. Conclusion: "The implications of these results are that calcium may play a substantial contributing role in reducing the incidence of obesity and prevalence of the insulin resistance syndrome."

Varenna, M.; Binell, L.; Casari, S.; Zucchi, F.; Sinigaglia, L.; *Effects of dietary calcium intake on body weight and prevention of osteoporosis in early postmenopausal women,* American Journal of Clinical Nutrition, 2007, September; 86(3): 639-44. A cross-sectional, retrospective, observational study of 1,771 healthy, early postmenopausal women. Conclusion: "BMI and prevalence of overweight showed significant inverse trends with increasing dairy intake."

Thorpe, M.P.; Jacobson, E.H.; Layman, D.K.; He, X.; Kris-Etherton, P.M.; Evans, E.M.; *A diet high in protein, dairy, and calcium attenuates bone loss over twelve months of weight loss and maintenance relative to a conventional high-carbohydrate diet in adults.* A randomized observation study of 130 overweight adult females and males for 12 months. Conclusion: "A reduced-energy diet supplying 1.4 g.kg(-1).d(-1) protein and 3 dairy servings increased urinary calcium excretion but provided improved calcium intake and attenuated bone loss over 4 mo. of weight loss and 8 additional mo of weight maintenance."

Zemel, M.B.; *The role of dairy foods in weight management.* Journal of the American College of Nutrition, 2005, December; 24(6 Suppl.): 537S-46S. A review and expert opinion. Conclusion: "These data indicate an important role for dairy products in both the ability to maintain a healthy weight and the management of overweight and obesity."

Designer milk

The capability to change the nutrient composition of our foods, including cow's milk, is only beginning to be appreciated.

The fact is, however, that we humans have been altering the nutrient composition of our available foods for several thousand years, through simple selection of preferred characteristics generation to generation, by cross-breeding and cross pollination, and through other forms of hybridization. But only recently have we been able to do so by modifying the genetic structure.

In the past, selection of preferred characteristics in our foods has been mostly directed to improving taste, usually by maximizing sweetness; increasing size and yield; and enhancing resistance to pests and predators. Little has been directed to improving the nutrient content. With good reason ... we simply didn't know much about our nutrient needs, and the nutrient content of our food choices. Plus, there has been a nagging complacency that concludes that the nutrients we need are readily available in ample quantities ... a complacency that is erroneously based and unjustified.

Givens, D.I.; *Session 4: Challenges facing the food industry in innovation for health. Impact on CVD risk of modifying milk fat to decrease intake of SFA and increase intake of cis-MUFA.* Proceeding of the Nutrition Society, 2008, November, 67(4): 419-27. Paper presented at symposium. Conclusion: "The present paper explores the options for replacing some of the SFA in milk fat with cis-MUFA through alteration of the diet of the dairy cow."

Henning, D.R.; Baer. R.J.; Hassan, A.N.; Dave, R.; *Major advances in concentrated and dry milk products, cheese, and milk-fat based spreads.* Journal of Dairy Science, 2008, April; 89(4): 1179-88. An expert statement. Conclusion: "Conjugated linoleic acid (omega-6), which can be increased in milkfat by alteration of the cow's diet, has been reported to have anticancer, anti-atherogenic, antidiabetic, and antiobesity effects for human health."

Hernandez, E.R.; Jacome, M.M.; Lee, R.G.; Nakano, T.; Ozimek, L. Guzman, I.V.; *High conjugated linoleic acid (CLA) content in milk and dairy products using a dietary supplementation of sunflower seed in cows. Thrombogenic/atherogenic risk issues.* Archivos Latinoamericanos de Nutricion, 2007, June; 57(2): 173-8. Controlled study. Conclusion: "...dietary supplementation of sunflower seed in cows increases the CLA and TVA (transvaccenic acid) content in milk, which may contribute to the reduction of the risk of cardiovascular diseases in humans."

Lopez-Huertas, E.; Teucher, B.; Boza, J.J.; Marinez-Ferez, A.; Majsak-Newman, G.; Baro, L.; Carrero, J.J.; Gonzalez-Santiago, M.; Fonolla, J.; Fairweather-Tait, S.; *Absorption of calcium from milks enriched with fructo-oligosaccharides, caseinophosphopeptides, tricalcium phosphate, and milk solids.* American Journal of Clinical Nutrition, 2006, February; 83(2): 310-6. Randomized, controlled, double-blind crossover study of fifteen volunteers. Conclusion: "Calcium-enriched milks are a valuable source of well-absorbed calcium. Absorption of added calcium as tricalcium phosphate was higher than that of calcium from the control milk."

Maubois, J.L.; *Milk and dairy products for human nutrition: contribution of technology.* Bulletin del Academie Nationale de Medecine (Paris), 2008, April, 192(4): 703-11. Expert comment. "The dairy industry is now able to offer consumers safe classical products (liquid milk, raw-milk cheeses) with little or no heat treatment. ....Combined with other separation technologies, membrane technologies should soon allow the separation and purification of minor milk proteins described as having essential roles in bone calcium uptake and vitamin transport, for example ...The use of enzymatic membrane reactors has led to the identification of several bioactive peptides, such as kappa-caseinomacropeptide, which induces CCK (cholecystokinin) secretion and thus regulates food intake and lipid assimilation, alpha(S1)CN (91-100), a compound with benzodiazepine activity, kappaCN (106-116), which has anti-thrombotic acivity by inhibiting blood platelet binding to fibrinogen, an alpha(S) and beta casein phophopeptides, which are thought to increase iron and calcium absorption."

Sabikhi, L.; *Designer milk,* Advances in Food and Nutrition Research, 2007, 53: 161-98. An expert opinion. Conclusion: "Modification of the primary structure of casein, alteration in the lipid profile, increased protein recovery, milk containing nutraceuticals, and replacement for infant formula offer several advantages in the area of processing.

49

Less fat in milk, altered fatty acid profiles, more protein, less lactose, and absence of beta-lactoglobulin (beta-LG) are some opportunities of 'designing' milk for human health benefits."

Steinshamn, H.; Purup, S.; Thuen, E.; Hansen-Moller, J.; *Effects of clover-grass silages and concentrate supplementation on the content of phytoestrogens in dairy cow milk.* Journal of Dairy Science, 2006, July, 91(7): 2715-25. Experimental study with 28 Norwegian Red dairy cows. Conclusion: "Overall, this study shows that feeding cows with silage containing red clover increases the milk content of flavonoids at both low and high concentrate supplementation levels."

References used in the text for Chapter Two

Aoki, T.; Aoe, S.; *Prevention of osteoporosis by foods and dietary supplements. Bioavailability of milk micellar calcium phosphate,* Clincal Calcium, 2006, October; 16(10): 1616-23.

Cook, A.J.; Friday, J.E.; *Food mixture of ingredient sources for dietary calcum: shifts in food group contributions using four grouping protocols,* Journal of the American Dietetic Association, Nov: 103(11): 1513-9, 2003.

Eaton, S.B., Nelson, D.A.; *Calcium in evolutionary perspective,* The American Journal of Clinical Nutrition, 54(1 Suppl): 281S-287S, July, 1991.

German, J.B.; Gibson, R.A.; Krauss, R.M.; Nestel, P.; Lamarche, B.; van Staversen, W.A.; Steijns, J.M.; de Groot, L.C.; Lock, A.L.; Destaillats, F.; *A reappraisal of the impact of dairy foods and milk fat on cardiovascular disease risk.* European Journal of Nutrition, 2009, June; 48(4): 191-203

Godbole, N.N. Dr.; *Milk, The Most Perfect Food,* Biotech Books, New Delhi, 2007. The quotation is from *Sushruta,* an English translation by Kavira Kunalal, vol. 1, 1907, pp 430-434.

Groff, James L.; Gropper, Sareen S.; Hunt, Sara M.; *Advanced Nutrition and Human Metabolism, Second Edition,* West Publishing Company, 1995

Gue'guen, Leon; Pointillart, MsSeAgr; Pointillart, Alain; *The Bioavailability of Dietary Calcium,* Journal of the American College of Nutrition, vol. 19, No. 90002, 119S-136S, 2000

Guthrie, Helen A.; Picciano, Mary Frances; *Human Nutrition,* Mosby, 1995.

International Dairy Foods Association, *The Importance of Milk in the Diet,* www.idfa.org/resource-center/industry-facts, 2009

Montgomery, M.R.; *A Cow's Life, The Surprising History of Cattle and How the Black Angus Came to be Home on the Range,* Walker & Company, 2004.

More, J.; *Children's bone health and meeting calcium needs,* Journal of Farm Health Care, 18(1):22-4, 2008

N.I.H., *PubMed Central (PMC),* U.S. National Institute of Healthe (N.I.H.), www.ncbi.nlm.nih.gov   PubMed is *the* source for biomedical articles, with access available to the public, comprising more than 19 million citations from MEDLINE and life science journals.

Scrimshaw, N.S.; Murray, E.B.; *The acceptability of milk and milk products in populations with a high prevalence of lactose intolerance,* American Journal of Clinical Nutrition, 48 Supplement: 1081-1159, 1988

Tortora, Gerald J.; Grabowski, Sandra Reynolds; *Principles of Anatomy and Physiology, Seventh Edition,* Harper Collins, 1993.

USDA: *United States Department of Agriculture, Nutient Database for Standard Reference.* Food composition data is taken from this reference and compared with the dietary reference intakes listed in the *USDA DRI Tables: Dietary Guidance: Food and Nutrition Information Center.* It should be noted that the USDA Food Composition Data Base is *the* primary reference source for the nutrient content of food, and is used worldwide. It is an extensive data base, with its beginnings dating back to 1891, when the first food composition tables were published by W.O Atwater and C.D. Woods, who assayed the refuse, water, fat, protein, ash, and carbohydrate content of 200 different foods. The current data base has data for more than 130 nutrients for 7,538 different foods, and is continually being expanded and updated. The data base is the reference for all of the nutrition soft-ware programs, such as Food Processor, the Nutritionist series, Nutri Genie, and Nutri Base, and for almost all scientific evaluations. Only a few years ago the data base provided information for only 9 vitamins and 9 minerals ... but now includes all of the 14 essential vitamins and 10 minerals. Still lacking, however, is data for the essential minerals chloride, sulphur, boron, arsenic, chromium, floride, molybdenum, nicked, silicon, vanadium, and iodine.

The food composition data base can be accessed on the internet at http://www.ars.usda.gov/nutrientdata, and the dietary reference intakes at http://www.nal.usda.gov/fnic .

Calculations of the nutrient composition of milk was carried out using these two references and then extrapolating values for an eight-ounce serving (8 ounces = 28.35 X 8 = 227 grams). The mean adult intake references were used for daily recommended intakes.

University of Guelph, *Introduction to Dairy Science and Technology: Milk History, Consumption, Production, and Composition;*2010 http://www.foodsci.uoguelph.ca/dairyedu/intro.html

Wikipedia, *Milk*, www.en.wikipedia.org/wiki/Milk

Wikipedia, *Dairy Cattle*, www.en.wikipedia.org/wiki/Dairy_cattle

Summary Statement for Chapter Two, the 'Good'

There is clearly a lot of 'good' to say about milk, and there have been an abundance of studies and observations to support the case for milk. In fact, the number of studies, strength of conclusions, and the test of time all combine to give the 'good' of milk substantial credibility. This cannot be ignored.

CHAPTER THREE

'THE BAD'

How long have we been drinking liquid cow's milk?

The story of how cow's milk became a favorite drink of American and other Western populations is a fascinating tale full of controversy and grand arguments both for and against. As I mentioned in the introduction chapter, humans did not succeed in domesticating the descendents of the giant primordial ox, the *auroch,* sufficiently to extract the milk from its udder until about 7,000 years ago. But drinking fluid milk in significant quantities did not become common until much later. Melanie DuPuis, in her delightful book, *Nature's Perfect Food,* reminds us that drinking fluid cow's milk did not really become popular in America until the mid-eighteen hundreds, and that there were several decades of bitter debate over whether or not it was advisable to drink it at all, even then. Prior to that time most cow's milk was consumed in fermented forms, or as cheese and other products. Beginning in the 1850s, fluid milk 'straight from the cow' became sought after primarily as a breast-milk substitute for infants and a beverage for weaned children. Dupuis explains that the historically unprecedented transition from breastfeeding to using cow's milk as a substitute was the result of a major shift during that era in women's perception of themselves and their bodies, plus the effects of urbanization and heightened socio-economic status. In addition, the availability, convenience, and low cost of milk made it an attractive food option for the rapidly expanding urban populations. But in those early years fluid milk, especially as it was aggressively produced for the burgeoning urban masses, such as in New York City, was unclean and the source of much ill health. The medical historian, P.J. Atkins, dubbed cow's milk as it was produced in the mid-eighteen-hundreds as "white poison". He provides historical evidence that the milk of the time "was heavily contaminated with bacteria and was responsible for spreading a variety of diseases such as scarlet fever and tuberculosis. Infants not wholly breastfed were particularly vulnerable to diarrheal infections. Improvements such as pasteurization and bottling were slow to spread and are unlikely to have had much impact before the 1920s." (Atkins, 1992)

Are our physiologies adapted for milk consumption?

S. Boyd Eaton and Melvin Konner introduced nutritional science to the concept that our physiologies are designed for a lifestyle and food supply that existed prior to the age of agriculture, which began approximately 10,000 years ago. They first published the results of their arduous and meticulous studies in the prestigious *New England Journal of Medicine* in 1985, followed with a book entitled *The Paleolithic Prescription* three years later. Some of their observations and conclusions were truly startling. For example, they noted that with the advent of agriculture humankind's height dropped six inches, and that the domestication of animals and food plants radically changed the nutrient quality of both food sources.

I was studying at the University of Hawaii when I first learned about their studies. I was intrigued, and dug into some intensive research to learn more about their discoveries. One thing that interested me was that it seemed like they had succeeded in catching the scientific community totally off-guard. Although their study was published in what is considered to be the most prestigious peer-review scientific journal in the U.S., there was virtually no response to their paper for four years ... neither in support nor in criticism ... and then there was only a trickle of references for several more years. They re-published a follow-up paper in 1997 in the European Journal of Clinical Nutrition, entitled *Paleolithic nutrition revisited: A twelve-year retrospective on its nature and implications.* From that stage on their studies have been much discussed and reviewed. For me it was a lesson in the scientific process ... a scientist's work may have been carried out in keeping with the highest standards, and their results and conclusions carefully and credibly presented, but peer review and acceptance by the scientific community may take a very long time to come about.

Although Eaton and Konner's work built on earlier studies, notably by the gastroenterologist, Walter L. Voegtlin (*The stone age diet: Based on in-depth studies of human ecology and the diet of man, 1975)*, they are credited with being the pioneers in this exciting new field of study. The subject of the Paleolithic diet is now a well-known and popular theme, and has also prompted a new field of medicine called "Evolutionary Medicine" (Trevathan, Smith, and McKenna, 1999).

The question which arises in context with this new understanding of our nutritional history and the adaptive design of our physiologies ... applied to the case of cow's milk ... is whether or not our modern-day physiologies are suited to the consumption of this relatively new food.

Eaton and Konner suggest that the answer is 'no' ... that the consumption of cow's milk is too recent an event for our physiologies to have genetically modified or adapted to accommodate this food, particularly as adults. The prevalence of lactose intolerance among various ethnic groups would be a supportive case in point for this conclusion. On the other hand, the apparent mutations that occurred with the Funnel Beak Culture and at least two early African populations suggest otherwise. The adaptation and dominance of light-colored skin among indigenous northern Europeans also supports the argument that yes, we *have* and *can* adapt to drinking cow's milk and consuming dairy products. More about lactose intolerance below.

The new anti-milk movement

The campaign to improve the quality of milk and to promote its production and consumption in the late 1800s and early 1900s is a huge success story, and milk drinking became firmly established as a typically American, or Western habit by the 1920s.

Despite the growing consumption of dairy products worldwide, however, a new aversion to drinking milk has emerged in recent years, beginning in the early 1970s. This has been the result of several factors and arguments, which, in addition to the historical perspective discussed above, can be summarized as follows:

1. With increased knowledge about our human nutrient needs and improved food composition data, the finding that cow's milk is lacking in many essential nutrients.

2. An emerging consensus among scientists and health care professionals that human breast milk is best for infants, and using cow's milk as a substitute should be discouraged.

3. A growing awareness that lactose intolerance is a real issue that cannot be ignored.

4. Awareness that recommendations to consume milk and dairy products is not politically correct, considering that most non-white ethnic groups are lactose intolerant, and evidence that calcium requirements for non-white ethnic groups may be different.

5. Vegetarians propose that we should not be eating animal-based foods for health reasons.

6. Animal rights groups argue that animals raised for food are abused and mis-treated, especially by big-business enterprises, and that perhaps we shouldn't be eating the flesh of other animal species for food.

7. A resistance by some people to purchase non-organic foods, or products produced by unscrupulous, overly profit orientated big business, with questionable quality and product composition.

8. Negative consumer reaction to the treatment of cow's with rBGH, anti-biotics, and other substances ... used to increase milk production.

9. The knowledge that commercial milk can be contaminated with blood, pus, manure, and more.

10. A reaction towards labeling laws that do not ensure that we know what is in the milk and milk products we consume ... plus concerns about false advertising.

11. The awareness of a possible contradiction between high calcium intake from dairy products and osteoporosis.

12. Accumulating scientific evidence linking cow's milk to a number of disease conditions in humans.

1. <u>Nutrient deficiencies</u>

Is it possible that 'nature's most perfect food' could be seriously lacking in some essential nutrients? Well, it is not only possible, but it is fact!

Vitamin C

Cow's milk has no vitamin C. The USDA Food Composition Data Base reports that 100 grams of whole cow's milk contains 0.0 milligrams of vitamin C. Is this surprising? What about the vitamin in cow's food? There is no data for the vitamin C content of field grasses, but the content in lemon grass is 2.6 mg per 100 grams. The two most used grain feeds are soybean and corn ... one hundred grams of raw soybeans contains only 6 mg of vitamin C, and 100 grams of raw sweet corn 6.8 mg. But even the little that is contained in the normal cow's food is apparently not transferred to its milk. This makes sense, however, when it is realized that the cow ... *and* its calf ... produces its own vitamin C. As mentioned elsewhere in this book, this is one of the curiosities of our human metabolism and a quirk of mother nature. All of the animals in the animal kingdom produce their own vitamin C, except, that is, for a tiny group which include humans, the gorilla and chimpanzee, the guinea pig, fruit bat, and one species of birds. We lack the last enzyme in the vitamin C synthetic pathway, *gulonolactone oxidase* . Yes, we are *that* close to completing the synthesis. (*Advanced Nutrition And Human Metabolism, 2005*) This fact suggests that at one time, earlier in our evolution, our ancestors *did* produce vitamin C, but that a negative mutation prevented the final step. It also suggests that the mutation took hold because our ancestors at that time lived in an environment so abundant in vitamin C that there was no need for us to make our own. Humans, therefore, must obtain this important essential nutrient in our food supply, but not the cow and almost all other animals. And therefore drinking milk cannot help us get enough of this vitamin.

Vitamin A and D

Milk is touted for its ability to give us the fat soluble vitamins A, especially vitamin D, and also vitamins E and K ... contained in the fat part of milk. Vitamin D is normally required for our bodies to absorb and utilize calcium, so it could be considered an essential component of milk, or essentially included in the diet, needed to utilize the calcium in milk. However, if the fat in milk is taken out, as with lowfat or skim milk, then these vitamins are taken out as well. Whole milk contains 104 mcg of vitamin A, 0.23 mcg of vitamin D, 160 mcg of vitamin E, and 0.7 mcg of vitamin K, in one eight-ounce glass, but only 32 mcg of vitamin A, 0 mcg of vitamin D, 0.02 mcg of vitamin E, and 0.23 mcg of vitamin K is contained in a glass of lowfat milk (1% fat). Even with whole milk, however, these vitamins are not well supplied: one 8-ounce glass of whole milk provides only 13% of your recommended vitamin A intake, 4.5 % vitamin D, 1.1% vitamin E, and 1.7% vitamin K. For lowfat milk these percentages drop to 4.0%, 0.0001%, 0.00001%, and 0.6%, repectively.

Iodine

The amount of iodine in cow's milk, taken from samples worldwide, cannot be detected by normal laboratory methods (Kikuchi, 2008).

The missing minerals ... iron, zinc, potassium, manganese, magnesium, and others

While cow's milk is rich in calcium and phosphorous, it does not fare so well in respect to several other minerals. An eight-ounce glass of milk, for example, provides only 1.5% of our daily requirement of iron, only 4.8% of our needed zinc, 4.4% of potassium, and 1.4% of our manganese. It notably lacks in another major mineral needed for bone maintenance, magnesium ... one glass supplying only 4.14% of our requirement. This is a much over-looked fact, which may explain part of the story why heavy milk-drinking populations still have high rates of osteoporosis. The ratio of recommended magnesium intake to calcium is 379 mg to 1000 mg. But 4 glasses of milk, providing 1,000 mg of calcium, only gives 90.8 mg of magnesium. Many feel that even this guideline ratio is too low ... some have suggested that a 2:1 ratio is more correct ... others have claimed even higher ratios yet, claiming that the role of magnesium has been grossly underestimated. Regardless, it is clear that milk does not provide sufficient amounts of magnesium to balance the calcium content.

Calcium, magnesium, and one other mineral, potassium, are also known to act as alkaline buffers in the body's acid-base balance homeostasis function. The low amounts of magnesium and potassium in milk contribute to milk and milk products' acid-producing property ... cheeses have the highest 'potential acid renal load' (PARL) of all foods, for example. More about this later in the chapter.

Other minerals lacking in milk are copper and selenium. The USDA Food Composition data base does not list the available amounts in milk for chloride, sulphur, arsenic, boron, chromium, floride, molydenum, nickel, silicon, and vanadium, so how milk fares in respect to these minerals is unknown. We do know, however, that cow's milk contains almost no boron or silicon, two minerals that are particularly essential to bone maintenance (Groff, 1995)

Fatty acids ... omega-3 ??

Another nutrient of concern is the essential fatty acid, linolenic acid, or 'omega-3'. We knew little of this substance, and the need for it, before we discovered that the Greenland Eskimos, who had copious amounts in their food supply, had no atherosclerosis or heart disease ... but could easily die from a nose bleed. We now know that this fatty acid, and the EPA and DHA that are the end products of its metabolic pathway, are critical for the maintenance of optimal health, especially in turning our metabolism away from excessive coagulation and inflammation, and such things as the formation of plaque in our arteries. Further, we now know that the metabolic pathway of the second essential fatty acid, linoleic acid, or 'omega 6' leads to araachadonic acid and an opposing metabolic pathway favoring an inflammation and coagulation response. We also know that there is no homeostatic, or 'automatic' function within our physiologies to regulate which of these two pathways is prioritized ... the end production of araachadonic acid versus EPA and DHA depends solely on the amounts of each essential fatty acid we ingest, whether it is omega-3 or omega-6, and the successful completion of their two separate pathways.

It is theorized that once-upon-a-time in our humanoid ancestry we must have spent a long time in an environment that was rich in both linoleic and linolenic essential fatty acids, and thus lost, or never developed, a homeostatic function to regulate their pathways. This could have been a jungle environment, full of a large variety of plants, or maybe even near an ocean or large lake. The lake area in East Africa could have been this environment. Regardless, it remains that we don't have a homeostatic function, and so we are at the mercy of our own food choices and amounts consumed.

We find, however, that we can 'cheat' if we ingest the EPA or DHA direct, as it is found in fish oil. However, we usually consume much more omega-6 in our diets, especially since the vastly increased consumption of vegetable oils in the form of margarines and cooking oils since we decided to drop using butter in favor of vegetable-based products after WWII. In addition, the availability of omega-3 has greatly diminished. Wild grains and plants *do* contain substantial amounts of linolenic acid, as does the flesh of animals that feed on these wild plants. But linolenic acid is almost non-existent in domesticated grains and plants, and the meat of animals that feed on these domesticated plants is also void of linolenic acid. As a result, there are very few good sources of omega-3 in our modern food supply. Among the vegetable oils only the oil of the rapeseed, or 'canola' oil, and soybean oil, has any appreciable amounts. Flaxseed has some. For any substantial amount of omega-3 we must therefore look to the end products of the pathway, EPA and DHA, found in the fatty oils of fish such as the salmon, cod, shrimp, tuna, mackerel, herring, and the King crab. In addition, the linolenic pathway is much more vulnerable to interruption ... by anti-oxidants, for example. It has been reported that an anti-oxidant presence equivalent to 250 mg of vitamin E will block the pathway.

There is also a major controversy about what *ratio* of omega-6 to omega-3 will optimize the health effect. Our current guidelines suggest a ratio of 13:1. There is considerable evidence to indicate that this ratio is greatly in error. S.B. Eaton and Melvin Konner, in their landmark studies of our ancenstral diets, find that the ratio in the diet of early man was very close to unity (1:1), and suggests that our physiologies are designed for that kind of ratio.

Much has been written about the value of milk in providing linoleic and linolenic acid. Cow's milk does have some amounts of these two essential fats, depending on the particular cow's feed, as discussed in the previous chapter. As noted, domesticated feed grains are notably lacking in linolenic acid, and so very little omega-3 ends up in the cow's milk. However, the USDA food composition data base indicates that an eight-ounce glass of whole milk will contain 0.27 grams of linoleic fat and 0.17 grams of linolenic fat. In lowfat milk the linoleic amount drops to 0.06 grams and the linolenic falls to 0.009 grams, which is because these two essential fatty acids are contained in the fat part of whole milk.

Regardless, the claim that milk provides ample amounts of either linoleic acid or linolenic acid does not hold ground. The USDA food composition data indicates that an 8-ounce glass of whole milk contains only 2% of the daily recommended amount of 13.5 grams of linoleic acid, and 12.6% of the recommended intake of 1.35 grams of linolenic acid (omega-3). However, the current NIH recommendations for the ratio of omega-6 to omega-3 intake is 13:1. If the recommended ratio of omega-6 to omega-3 were to follow Eaton and Konner's recommended 1:1, then that eight-ounce glass of milk would provide only 1.2% of our needed omega-3 essential fatty acid

The conclusion, then, is that cow's milk is a poor source for much needed essential fatty acids, especially omega 3.

Quality of milk protein … a different point of view

In the previous chapter I discussed the pro side of milk protein. Casein protein and whey protein are both considered to be complete proteins, and according to the Protein Digestibility Corrected Amino Acid Score (PDCAAS) method of evaluating proteins, milk proteins are given the highest score (1.0). This is the method adopted by both the U.S. FDA the World Health Organization (FAO/WHO). This method is based on each protein's contribution to growth, especially among children, and this is the reason why the method is preferred by FAO/WHO … it is more useful in the context of international situations and particularly with developing countries. The FDA followed suit in this respect and adopted the same preferred measurement of quality as the FAO/WHO.

It was decided in a FAO/WHO meeting back in 1990 that proteins having values higher than 1.0 would be rounded down to 1.0. So … then

... do any proteins have a higher value than milk protein? The answer is yes. One is egg protein. Despite what you hear at the health food store or from bodybuilders, egg protein has the highest quality rating and is still the standard by which to measure other proteins. Digestibility of egg protein is 97% and the bioavailability is 94%. This means that we utilize 94% of the egg protein, and that in turn tells us that this composition of amino acids is at least 94% of the *most optimal* composition. Casein and whey proteins run a close second, especially whey protein, but egg protein still comes out on top.

More importantly, however, the milk proteins are not as 'complete' as egg protein. Over-all, milk protein is 'limiting' in the sulfur-containing amino acids, methionine and cysteine. For example, it is known that the combination of milk with legumes (which lack methionine) does not provide a complete protein (Gropper, 2005). Others report that milk is also limiting in tryptophan and lysine.

A story to tell

I have a story to tell. The omega-3 controversy was a central pet-peeve of our biochemistry professor at UH, and he spent much effort stressing the importance of the new findings. It was about the year 1996, and a major symposium on fats in general was being held at the East-West Center, and our professor was invited to speak on omega-3. He did so, and the next day in class he was long-faced and deeply troubled. He related to us what had happened. He said something like this: "Here was a group of the most prestigious nutritionists in the U.S., and some from other countries ... and what I told them fell on deaf ears. There was no response to my lecture ... not even questions! When I took one nutritionist aside afterwards, asking why the negative reaction, she remarked, 'How can we take this seriously? You are telling us that we have to tell Americans to eat fish ... but most Americans don't eat fish!'"

A case in point: India's predicament

It is interesting that the nation that produces the most milk for human consumption and supports its use through ancient literature and religious scriptures, is also the country that has the worst record of nutritional well-being. Although India has developed numerous programs to combat its nutritional problems ... since independence over 60 years ago ... the nation's nutritional status is appalling, and worsening. Its third National Family Health Survey, 2005-06, highlighted its many health issues. For example, India ranked the highest with undernutrition-among-children-under-five-years-of-age among 41 developing countries surveyed by the World Health Organization (WHO) between 2003 and 2007. Astonishingly, 48% of India's under-fives are chronically malnourished, which is almost twice as high as the average prevalence for sub-Saharan African countries. One in every three malnourished childen in the world lives in India. Thirty-six percent of adult women and 34 percent of men are undernourished. Among the Indian well-to-do overweight and obesity are emerging problems, with 13% of women and 9% of men either overweight or obese. The three most prevalent and most serious nutrient deficiencies are iron, iodine, and vitamin A. Seven out of every 10 children in India are anemic. More than half of women (55%) and almost one-quarter of men (24%) are anemic. An estimated 167 million people in India are at risk of iodine deficiency, of whom 54 million have goiter, and over 8 million have neurologic handicaps as a result of the lack of iodine (Biswas, 2002, Ramji, 1995, WHO, 1997). The prevalence of vitamin A deficiency was calculated to be 30.8% nationwide in 2002 (West, 2002)

Statistics compiled by the International Osteoporosis Foundation indicate that India also has a severe problem with osteoporosis. In a recent publication entitled *Facts and statistics about osteoporosis and its impact,* their concluding summary for India states: "In a study among Indian women aged 30-60 years from low income groups, BMD at all the skeletal sites were much lower than values reported from developed countries, with a high prevalence of osteopenia (52%) and osteoporosis (29%) thought to be due to inadequate nutrition." (IOF, 2010)

It is unfair, however, to propose that India's nutritional problems are due to simply drinking milk, because the roots of the country's health predicament are various, and go far beyond favoring milk as one food choice. The most critical factor is probably India's very high rate of population growth. The nation's population passed the one billion mark in March of 2001, and was estimated to be 1.17 billion in July, 2009, making it the most populous country on earth, second only to China. But with a birth rate of 22 per thousand, it is projected that India's population will surpass China's by about the year 2030. With 17.5% of the world's population and only 2.4% of the earth's land mass, India's peoples are caught between a rock and a very hard place ... a burgeoning population with limited resources.

It should be noted that more than half of the animal milk production is from the *water buffalo*, not the conventional cow. Although, the milk of the buffalo is considered to be very similar to that of the cow, there are significant differences. The following table outlines the most notable dissimilarities, based on a single 8-ounce serving of whole milk

Table 1: Comparison of cow and buffalo milk

	Cow's Milk	%RDA	Buffalo Milk	%RDA
Energy (kcal)	138.5		220.2	
Protein (g)	7.2	14%	8.5	16.7%
Fat	3.27		6.89	
Saturated fat (g)	4.23		4.6	
Calcium (mg)	256.5	25.6%	383.6	38.4%
Iron (mg)	0.068	1.52%	0.272	2.1%
Magnesium (mg)	22.7	4.1%	70.37	19.0%
Manganese	0.0091	1.4%	0.041	3.7%
Phosphorous (mg)	190.7	27.2%	265.6	37.9%
Potassium (mg)	299.6	4.4%	404.6	8.6%
Zinc (mg)	0.84	8.8%	0.50	5.3%
Iodine (mcg)	non-detectable		non-detectable	
Vitamin C (mg)	0	0%	5.22	6.3%
Vitamin A (mcg, RAE)	104.4	13.05%	120.3	15.0%
Pantothenic acid (mg)	0.847	16.9%	0.44	8.8%
Vitamin B-6 (mg)	0.082	4.3%	0.052	4.0%
Lysine (amino acid, g)	0.311		0.636	
Methionine (amino acid, g)	0.166		0.220	
Cystine (amino acid, g)	0.036		0.109	

A review of the values in this table point out some very interesting facts, and comparisons. First of all, this shows that both cow's milk and buffalo milk do not offer any help with India's first two nutrient deficiencies, namely iron, a lack of which cause anemia, and iodine. An 8 ounce glass of cow's milk provides 0.068 milligrams of iron, or only 1.52 % of our RDA. The same serving of buffalo's milk contains three times that amount, but this still only amounts to 2.6% of our RDA. Further, there is so little iodine in both cow's milk and buffalo milk that it cannot be detected by normal laboratory assays (Kikuchi, 2008).

It is interesting, in addition, that buffalo milk has 50% more calcium, over 3 times as much magnesium, 35% more potassium, significantly more of the sulfur-containing amino acids (methionine and cystine), and actually provides some vitamin C.

2. **Designed for cows, not humans**

Since the year 1971, when the practice of breastfeeding reached an all-time low in America, there has been a growing consensus in the medical profession that cow's milk should *not* be fed to infants. In 1984 the office of the U.S. Surgeon General initiated the landmark "Surgeon General's Workshop on Breastfeeding" which delineated six priority breastfeeding issues and organized numerous events and actions. Their motto, "to protect, promote, and support breastfeeding" was championed by many other agencies and organizations in following years.

The current policy statements of representatives of the professional health care community, such as the American Academy of Family Physicians (AAFP), the American Academy of Pediatrics (AAP), and the American Dietetic Association are consistent with the conclusion that human milk is best for human babies. The AAFP policy statement is as follows:

"Breastmilk offers medical and psychological benefits not available from human milk substitutes. The AAFP recommends that all babies, with rare exceptions, be breastfed and/or receive expressed human milk exclusively for the first six months of life. Breastfeeding should continue with the addition of complementary foods throughout the second half of the first year. Breastfeeding beyond the first year offers considerable benefits to both mother and child, and should continue as long as mutually desired. Family physicians should have the knowledge to promote, protect, and support breastfeeding. (1989) (2007)"

Statements outlining the American Academy of Pedriatrics policy are consistent with the AAFP positon:

"Breastfeeding is the physiological norm for both mothers and their children. Breastmilk offers medical and psychological benefits not available from human milk substitutes. The AAFP recommends that all babies, with rare exceptions, be breastfed and/or receive expressed human milk exclusively for the first six months of life. Breastfeeding should continue with the addition of complementary foods throughout the second half of the first year. Breastfeeding beyond the first year offers considerable benefits to both mother and child, and should continue as long as mutually desired. Family physicians should have the knowledge to promote, protect, and support breastfeeding. (1989) (2007)." " Human milk is the preferred feeding for all infants, including premature and sick newborns, with rare exceptions. The ultimate decision on feeding of the infant is the mother's. Pediatricians should provide parents with complete, current information on the benefits and methods of breastfeeding to ensure that the feeding decision is a fully informed one. When direct breastfeeding is not possible, expressed human milk, fortified when necessary for the premature infant, should be provided."

The American Dietetic Association also endorses breastfeeding:

"It is the position of the American Dietetic Association that exclusive breast-feeding provides optimal nutrition and health protection for the first 6 months of life and breastfeeding with complementary foods from 6 months until at least 12 months of age is the ideal feeding pattern for infants. Breastfeeding is an important public health strategy for improving infant and child morbidity and mortality, and improving maternal morbidity, and helping to control health care costs."

Numerous other organizations have followed suit, which include the American Public Health Association and the World Alliance for Breastfeeding Action (WABA).

One reason why cow's milk is considered to be unsuited for human infants is because of its high *casein* content and low *whey* content, which can put a strain on an infant's immature digestive organs, notably the kidneys, and for this reason is not recommended before the age of 12 months. In addition, because the infant intestine is not properly equipped to digest non-human milk, diarrhea, intestinal bleeding, and the non-absorption of nutrients may result.

It is also important to note that cow's milk is the basis of almost all commercial infant formulas, the soy-based formulas being one exception. To reduce the negative effect of cow's milk in commercially prepared formulas, the milk is processed. This processing includes steps to make milk protein more easily digestible and to alter the whey-to-casein protein balance to a ratio closer to that of human milk, plus the addition of several essential ingredients (fortification), and/or the partial or total replacement of dairy fat with fats of vegetable or marine origin.

It is interesting that both the AAFP and the AAP do not directly discriminate against cow's milk … their policy wording is careful not to mention cow's milk ... although the intended meaning is clearly to avoid the use of cow's milk in infant feeding. As Dr. Frank Oski, the renowned pediatrician, explained in *Don't Drink Your Milk*:

"Among physicians, so much concern has been voiced about the potential hazards of cow milk that the Committee on Nutrition of the prestigious American Academy of Pediatrics, the institutional voice of practicing pediatricians, released a report entitled, 'Should Milk Drinking by Children Be Discouraged?' Although the Academy's answer to this question has (as of this writing) been a qualified 'maybe', the fact that the question was raised at all is testimony to the growing concern about this product, which for so long was viewed as sacred as the proverbial goodness of mother and apple pie." (1977)

3. <u>Lactose intolerance</u>

Most Americans and people from heavy milk-drinking areas such as northern and middle Europe, and Canada, Australia, and New Zealand, do not realize that in many parts of the world drinking cow's milk is uncommon and even considered to be repulsive. The *World Dairy Map, 2009*, put out by the International Farm Comparison Network (IFCN) shows that per capita milk consumption is less than 30 liters per year for most of South America, almost all of central and southern Africa countries, all of South East Asia, in other Asian countries such as Japan, Korea, and Taiwan, and is less than 6 liters for all of vast China. Marvin Harris, in his delightful book, *Good To Eat, Riddles of Food and Culture,* explains that most Asians are either indifferent about drinking milk, or, like the Chinese, have a cultural and historical aversion to drinking milk or consuming dairy products. Harris quotes the famous anthropologist, Robert Lowie:

"The Chinese and other eastern and Southeast Asian peoples do not merely have an aversion to the use of milk, they loathe it intensely, reacting to the prospect of gulping down a nice, cold glass of the stuff much as Westerners might react to the prospect of a nice, cold glass of cow saliva." (pp 130)

The explanation for this disparity of milk consumption worldwide is complex. It has a lot to do with lactose intolerance, or the other side of the same coin, 'lactase deficiency', and the historical and evolutionary process that enabled some populations to comfortably digest large amounts of cow's milk, while others cannot digest the complex sugar in milk, lactose, at all. The molecular structure of lactose is too large and complex to pass through the walls of the small intestine, and must be broken down to the simple sugars (monosaccharides) of glucose and galactose before passing through the wall membranes and being absorbed into the blood. The transformation of lactose into glucose and galactose depends on the availability of the enzyme *lactase*. Adult humanoids do not formulate this enzyme as part of their *normal* adult metabolism ... if they do, it is an *abnormal* condition, present in only a few of the many variations of human physiologies.

The molecular basis of lactose intolerance still eludes a precise explanation. Campbell et al theorizes that "two polymorphisms in the introns of a helicase upstream from the lactase gene correlate closely with hypolactasia, and thus lactose intolerance". He estimates that 4 billion of the world's population of 6.7 billion, or 60%, are genuinely lactose intoleranct. (Campbell, 2009)

A review in Wikipedia offers an excellent summary of the history and genetic prevalence of lactose intolerance:

"Lactose intolerance has been studied as an aid in understanding ancient diets and population movement in prehistoric societies. Milking an animal vastly increases the calories that may be extracted from the animal, as compared to the consumption of its meat alone. It is not surprising, then, that consuming milk products became an important part of the agricultural way of life in the Neolithic.

Roman authors recorded that the people of northern Europe, particularly Britain and Germany, drank unprocessed milk. This corresponds with modern European distributions of lactose intolerance, where the people of Britain, Germany and Scandinavia have a good tolerance, and those of southern Europe, especially Italy, have a poorer tolerance.

In east Asia, historical sources also attest that the Chinese did not consume milk, whereas the nomads that lived on the borders did. Again, this reflects modern distributions of intolerance. China is particularly notable as a place of poor tolerance, whereas in Mongolia and the Asian steppes horse milk is drank regularly. This tolerance is thought to be advantageous, as the nomads did not settle down long enough to process mature cheese or other milk products. Given that their prime source of income is generated through horses, to ignore their milk as a source of calories would probably have been detrimental. The nomads also make an alcoholic beverage, called Kumis, from horse milk ... the fermentation process reduces the amount of lactose present.

The African Fulani also have a nomadic origin and their culture once completely revolved around cow, goat, and sheep herding. Dairy products were once a major source of nutrition for them. As might be expected, lactase persistence evolved in response to dairy product consumption, and they are particularly tolerant to lactose (about 77% of the population). Many of Fulani origin live in Guinea-Conakry, Burkina Faso, Mali, Nigeria, Niger, Cameroon, and Chad.

There is some debate on exactly where and when genetic mutation(s) worldwide occurred, although a recent study suggests that the genetic change that enabled early Europeans to drink milk without getting sick had appeared in dairying farmers who lived around 7,000 years ago in a region between the central Balkans and central Europe (the Funnel Beaker Culture). Others have argued that separate mutation events occurred even earlier in Sweden (which has one of the lowest levels of lactose intolerance in the world) and in the Arabian Peninsula (around 4000 BC). However, others argue for a single mutation event in the Middle East at about 4500 BC, which then subsequently radiated. Some sources suggest a third and more recent mutation took place among the East African Tutsi. The Maasai, another group, possess the ability to consume dairy without exhibiting symptoms as well, but this may be due to a different genetic mutation or it may be due to the fact that they curdle their milk before they consume it, which removes the lactose.

Robert Holloway, in his study entitled *The Ancient Roots of Milk Consumption and its Genetic Dependence,* concludes that the earliest human population to raise cattle and consume milk products was the "Funnel Beaker Culture" of Northern Europe. Not only were they the first to consume milk, he states, but they were the only people to be genetically equipped to produce the enzyme lactase in adulthood ... and that all succeeding populations, at least in northern Europe, that became lactase sufficient acquired this genetic variation through inter-breeding, going back to the Funnel Beaker culture. Due to genetic dispersion over the centuries, lactase sufficiency varies ... it is not a case of either having it or not having it, but rather more a case of a degree of sufficiency. Holloway has compiled an informative scale of the "percent tolerance" among the peoples of 20 countries, as follows:

Table 2: Prevalence of lactose intolerance by country

Country	Percent Tolerance	Country	Percent Tolerance
Sweden	99%	Finland	82
Ireland	98	France	77
Denmark	97	Portugal	66
Netherlands	95	Poland	63
United Kingdom	95	India	50
United States	89	Greece	47
Swziterland	88	Italy	28
Austria	87	Mexico	17
Germany	85	Japan	10
Spain	85	China	7

Holloway goes on to draw a correlation between lactose percent tolerance and per capita consumption. The correlation is convincing.

Whatever the precise origin in time and place, most modern Northern Europeans and people of India, as well as people of European or Indian ancestry, show the effects of this mutation, while most modern East Asians, sub-Saharan Africans and native peoples of America and the Pacific Islands do not, making them lactose intolerant as adults.

Another story

At this point I must tell a story ... about lactose intolerance and my studies at University of Hawaii. During one of our undergraduate nutrition classes we were covering the lactose intolerance issue. Our professor, of Northern European ancestry and well doctrined in the conventional wisdom, was telling us that only a few peoples of the world were 'lactose intolerant' and could not drink milk. But the students at UH are an international and inter-racial mix, and several of the students disagreed. One stuck up her hand, and declared that 'most Asians are lactose intolerant'. Hmmm, sighed our teacher, "Yes, I think you are right". Another hand poked up, "Most blacks are also lactose intolerant !!" Another hmm. Then another, "Native Americans are lactose intolerant too !!" Our teacher was becoming worried. Yet another voice spoke out, "And that includes almost all the people in South America !!" Our professor gave a final sigh, and concluded, "Well, I guess that most of the people in the world are lactose intolerant ... it is only those of Northern European ancestry that are not."

A story of my own ... lactose intolerance and diabetes

It happened when I was fourteen, in the year of 1957. Our family had just moved up from the small town of Cardston in Southern Alberta to the thriving metropolis of Edmonton, and mom had just returned from a visit to the doctor with my baby sister, Wendy. Wendy had suffered from a hay fever condition since infancy, and we had just discovered that the reason for her slow development in speech and other things was because her sinuses were so plugged up that her hearing was seriously impaired ... and the doctor had diagnosed her condition as an allergy, with the probable cause being cow's milk. Wendy had been a bottle-fed baby, and had been consuming cow's milk from birth. Mom was furious, and I remember her storming through the house, announcing to us all in no uncertain terms that "this family will no longer drink milk" !!

But the problem with milk went beyond Wendy's allergy condition. Kathryn Fletcher had suffered from Type I diabetes since a young girl. Her appendix was removed when she was six, and the wound had refused to heal ... she missed a full year of school as a result. But Kathryn was a bright girl, and quickly made up her lost year, and gained another one, graduating from high school at seventeen, and then studied nursing at the Holy Cross Hospital in Calgary. She was determined to find a solution to her diabetes, and thought that she could find the answer by studying medicine. But she had become terribly disappointed ... conventional medicine had little to offer in her pursuit of a cure for her diabetes, and in those days little was understood about the connection between diet and diabetes ... at least within the conventional wisdom. And her condition was worsening. I remember a time when we were still in Cardston ... we were a poor family, with mom working in our retail shoe store, and dad on the road most of the time as a travelling salesman ... and mom's insulin was expensive, and so she sometimes went without it. I remember her being rushed to the hospital early one Sunday morning, hemorrhaging profusely.

Mom Bateman had a close, dear friend who had studied nursing with her, but who was also disillusioned with mainstream medicine, and had moved to Ogden, Utah, to open a 'health food store'. Her name was Betsy Shaeffer, a wonderful lady with a grand heart ... and a pioneer, for health foods was a novel idea in those days. I would know her later as my sweetheart's landlady, when I attended Weber State College in 1967. Kathryn Bateman decided to quit nursing and explore the mysterious world of health foods. She went to live and study with Betsy for a time, and then returned to Edmonton and worked in a tiny health food store on

Whyte Avenue, near the corner of 109th Street. This was all happening about the same time as the discovery that Wendy's allergy problem was probably linked to milk, and mom was being exposed to a lot of fresh ideas about diet and health, and how she could possibly control her diabetes ... and, even back then, there was strong suspicion that there was a connection between drinking cow's milk and the onset of diabetes.

It is unfortunate that Kathryn Fletcher's experience wasn't studied in a scientific way, because it seems that she fit all the conditions for a classic study of the association of cow's milk and diabetes ... and Wendy's allergy ... in fact, our whole family could have been an excellent study. You see, both sides of my family go back to Pennsylvania and dairy farming. My father once bragged that we were 'pure Pennsylvanian Dutch', on both sides. But my father's side had switched to grain farming when they had pioneered to Alberta, whereas Kathryn Fletcher's family had stuck to dairy farming, although my grandfather had also been a lawyer and a judge.

He was a 'hunchback' having suffered a twisted spine from a farm accident as a young boy ... then studied law in California, and became a judge in the small town of Burdett in Southern Alberta at the age of 33. He was a remarkable man, and greatly loved for his wisdom and high thinking. The Blood Indian tribe had made him an honorary chief ... I remember seeing his magnificent headdress of feathers and finely crafted leather among my mother's chest of treasures ... and I was presented with a gift of wonderfully crafted leather moccasins when I was in Cardston, and my mother had taken me to a Blood Indian pow-wow. They called my mother 'the daughter of Mister Fletcher'.

We were all lactose intolerant. And to no small degree. We used to joke among ourselves that mom was 'gas powered'. But myself as well. One glass of milk used to do it. Even now I need to be careful. And yet I love milk. A bowl of oatmeal porridge or cornflakes without milk is unthinkable. And in the years before mom made her grand declaration, all of us drank a lot of milk. Coming from a dairying background, mom had always thought milk to be the best of foods, and it was inexpensive and readily available ... and we were poor ... so she had encouraged us to drink milk as much as possible. We had it with our cereal in the mornings, and with a full glass or two as well, and our most common mid-day meal was good 'ol Campbell's tomato soup, diluted with, of course, milk. I think I must have had tomato soup for lunch for well over half of the time during those days. Tomato soup and milk ... with whole-wheat bread broken up and added to the soup !! We were definitely *not* a gourmet family. And gas !? ... well, we just thought it was kinda normal.

Yes, we would have all made a grand study. On my father's side everyone was hearty and lived long. My father's father lived to be 94, and, as my father put it, he only died because he decided to. But on my mother's side ... well ... everyone died early of stroke and heart disease, and diabetes was common. My grandfather, the judge, died at 36, of heart attack. One uncle had gone AWOL at D-Day in Normandy, but had died of a heart attack on a dance floor shortly after, barely having reached his thirtieth birthday. Mom lasted much longer than most, but died at 72 with her second stroke. I have already had my first stroke, and am probably living on borrowed time. It is likely that I had advanced atherosclerosis even as a youngster.

An interesting complication to the lactose intolerance problem is that some processed foods and beverages contain added lactose sugar without this fact being revealed on the label. (Campbell, 2009) This can lead to lactose intolerance symptoms without the person even being aware that they have ingested lactose. Food products that may contain lactose include:
- Bread and other baked goods
- Processed breakfast cereals
- Instant potatoes, soups, and breakfast drinks
- Margarine
- Lunch meats (other than kosher)
- Salad dressings
- Candies and other snacks
- Mixes for pancakes, biscuits, and cookies

(Medhelp, 2010)

4. Lactose intolerance: can it be treated ... and are dairy intake recommendations politically correct ?

There has been a great deal written about lactose intolerance as a treatable and abnormal condition. The problem has been down-played by even the World Health Organization (WHO) and giants in the international field of nutrition such as Nevin Schrimshaw. The intent is clear, and is honorable ... major international health agencies and professionals in health and nutrition view animal milk as a valued and much needed addition to food sources for high risk populations in developing countries. There is a similar concern in the U.S., and lactose intolerance is purposefully down-played. But there is a more recent awareness that these good intentions should go only so far, and the problem of lactose intolerance is real and cannot be ignored. It can also be considered politically incorrect when assuming that all populations can benefit from milk consumption.

Melanie DuPuis, in *Nature's Perfect Food,* pulls no punches when she states:

> "The privileged discourse about the perfection of milk has left out those people – mostly people of color – who are genetically lactose-intolerant. The perfect whiteness of this food and the white body genetically capable of digesting it in large quantities become linked. By declaring milk perfect, white northern Europeans announced their own perfection." (pp 11)

Elsewhere she adds:

> "The establishment of white racial hegemony and the celebration and purification of a white substance digested predominantly by this group become more than accidental." (pp 14)

A racial bias in the U.S. national nutrition policy has been noted. The Physicians Committee for Responsible Medicine published a statement addressing this issue as far back as 1999. The abstract summarizes their statement as follows:

> "The Dietary Guidelines for Americans form the basis for all federal nutrition programs and incorporate the Food Guide Pyramid, a tool to educate consumers on putting the Guidelines into practice. The Pyramid recommends two or three daily servings of dairy products. However, research has shown that lactase nonpersistence, the loss of enzymes that digest the milk sugar lactose, occurs in a majority of African-, Asian-, Hispanic-, and Native American individuals. Whites are less likely to develop lactase nonpersistence and less likely to have symptoms when it does occur. Calcium is available in other foods that do not contain lactose. Osteoporosis is less common among African Americans and Mexican Americans than among whites, and there is little evidence that dairy products have an effect on osteoporosis among racial minorities. Evidence suggests that a modification of federal nutrition policies, making dairy-product use optional in light of other calcium sources, may be a helpful public measure." (Berton et al, 1999)

A review of the most recent guidelines for Americans published by the United States Department of Agriculture (USDA) and the Food and Nutrition Information Center (FNIC) indicates that alternatives to dairy products are now being offered.

A few studies have found an increased association of milk consumption with certain disease conditions among individuals who are lactose intolerant. This makes sense when one considers that the negative impact on well-being when a person who is lactase insufficient ingests lactose can exert additional stress on the body and metabolism. Shrier et al (2008), for example, applied statistical analysis to subjects who were separated into two groups: either lactase persistent (LP) or lactase nonpersitent (LNP), and tested for associations with a number of disease conditions. Significant differences were noted. Interestingly, while the risk for stomach cancer increased with the lactose intolerant group, the risk decreased with prostate, ovarian, and breast cancers, and even suggested protection against colorectal cancer. This may suggest that the ability to digest lactose increases the risk for this latter group of diseases. I examine this concept in more detail in the "association with disease" section later in this chapter.

An interesting complication to the lactose intolerance problem is that some processed foods and beverages contain added lactose sugar without this fact being revealed on the label. (Campbell, 2009) This can lead to lactose intolerance symptoms without the person even being aware that they have ingested lactose.

A final story about lactose intolerance

While studying at the University of Mahidol one of our *ajaan* (professors) told about when she was involved in an international assistance effort with refugees fleeing from the Cambodian Khmer Rouge during the late 1970s. A large number of infants and children were being rescued and were receiving treatment at border hospital camps set up by international aid groups, mostly American. The young victims were severely malnourished, showing visible signs of *kwashiorkor and marasmus* and many were near death. The American doctors began to feed these infants and children powdered milk, assuming that this was the best possible food for them. A large percentage of them immediately reacted with increased diarrhea, becoming even more malnourished and ill, and even dying. The Thai Department of Health sent in a team of Thai doctors and nutritionists, my ajaan one of them, to diplomatically explain to the American doctors that the Cambodian Kmer were naturally lactose intolerant, and their young children could not digest cow's milk ... the American doctors were killing them by feeding them powdered cow's milk !!

Another aspect of the political correctness issue that should be included is the evidence that non-white ethnic groups do not need the same high levels of calcium intake, and therefore recommendations for dairy intake based on calcium requirements for those of Northern European ancestry may not apply. This evidence comes from studies of the incidence of osteoporosis, and the finding that although non-white groups tend to consume less dairy, due to lactose intolerance, and therefore obtain less calcium in their diets, they consistently demonstrate lower rates of osteoporosis. This is covered further in the section on osteorporosis.

5. <u>The vegetarian point of view</u>

Vegetarians, at least vegans, do not drink milk or consume dairy products on the grounds that they are derived from animals ... it is not a plant food. This, then, is surely a reason why I should embrace their point of view as support for the position that we should not drink milk. However, I find it hard to do so enthusiastically because much of their reasoning and conclusions are based on flawed science, illogical reasoning, and an almost religious zeal. In this section and also in the section on calcium and osteoporosis, I therefore put forward their arguments as support for the case why we shouldn't drink milk, but I also present evidence that counters their conclusions.

Vegetarianism has been around forever, it seems. Walter Gratzer, in his highly entertaining *Terrors of the Table, A Curious History of Nutrition* (Gratzer, 2005), tells us about the many variations and different movements of vegetarianism throughout history, beginning with the mathematician and philosopher, Pythagoras, of early Greece ... his name later revered by one group of 19th century vegetarians, calling themselves 'Pythagoreans'. The Hindus, Jains, Zoroastrians, and modern day Seventh-Day-Adventists all embraced or still embrace vegetarianism.

During my days of youth, spending much time working in my mother's health food store, vegetarianism seemed to be in-thing in Canada and America, and was promoted by a number of writers and nutrition 'gurus'. Then there seemed to be a lapse in enthusiasm for the fad, until the early 80's. John McDougall wrote his *The McDougall Plan* in 1983, John Robbins published *Diet For A New America* in '87, and a new enthusiasm seemed to emerge. Dean Ornish, although not really pushing vegetarianism, contributed to the movement with *Dr. Dean Ornish's Program for Reversing Heart Disease* in 1990 and *Eat More, Weigh Less* in 1993. John Robbins followed with a second book, *The Food Revolution,* published in 2001. Each of these authors contribute to a better understanding of our nutrition options, and Robbins in particular underscores the appeal to end our dependence on animal foods and the obscenities of raising and butchering animals on a large, big-business scale, with much cruelty dealt to the animals. However, it must also be noted that the writings by these authors demonstrate a strong bias towards vegetarianism, and sometimes draw on questionable research and reach invalid conclusions. One example involves the subject of osteoporosis, which I deal with in greater detail later in this chapter. I also explore these books in depth in another part of *The Nutrition Factor: A Bold New Perspective.*

There are several variations of the vegetarian option. Some persons choose to exclude only red meats, and will therefore still consume fish, dairy products, eggs, and poultry. Others go to the next step, and add poultry and fish to the list of unacceptable food choices, but will still consume dairy products and eggs ... these persons are called *lacto-ovo-vegetarians.* The *lacto-vegetarian* is then one that consumes only plants and dairy products. The hard-core vegetarian who consumes only plant foods is the *vegan.* When it comes to the exclusion of milk and milk products from the diet, this then refers only to the vegan.

There are not, however, many true vegans around. An article by Charles Stahler in the *Vegetarian Journal* cites the results of a 2006 national poll conducted by The Vegetarian Resource Group, indicating that only 1.4% of American men, and 1.3% of women are vegans, with 2.3% being vegetarian in a broader sense. I could not find worldwide statistics for vegans, but those classified in the wider definition of vegetarians showed that, except for India and Israel, the percentage of the adult population who were vegetarians ranged from a high of 4.3% for the Netherlands to a low of 1.5% for the Czech Republic. Israel has boasted that 8.5% of their adult population is vegetarian, while the vegetarian option in India accounts for 40%, or 399 million people. (Raw Food Health, 2010) It is not known what portion of these vegetarians do not consume milk or dairy products ... are true vegans. Since milk consumption in India is very high, for example, it can be surmised that they are mostly lacto-vegetarian in that country.

Should we pursue a vegetarian diet ?

This brings us to the question of whether or not we *should* pursue a vegetarian diet. This controversial question is relevant to the milk issue ... true vegans do not consume cow's milk, on the grounds that it is derived from an animal source, not a vegetable source.

This then, suggests a first counter- argument to the vegan's logic ... cow's milk is not the actual flesh of an animal, it is only the secretion of its mammalian glands ... much the same scenario as feeding milk from a human mother's breasts. Is drinking the milk of the cow, then, the same as eating meat?

Throughout my years studying nutrition in an academic setting, the issue of vegetarianism was carefully skirted and rarely addressed openly. I surmised that this was due to a couple of factors. One is that a good percentage of university students, especially girls, support the vegetarian logic, and try to be vegetarians themselves. Another is, I suspect, that we all, somewhere down deep inside, agree that we shouldn't be eating the flesh and products of other animals ... we are taking the life of other species in order to sustain ourselves.

A story about 'taking life' ...

It was the summer of '93, and I was attending a Natural Foods Convention being held in Las Vegas. There were a large number of lectures and debates being featured, and Dr. Jonathan White was a favorite speaker. I had already taken in several of the lectures, and couldn't help noticing one individual in particular. He was a small man, with black curly hair and was carefully manicured in a perfectly tailored suit, and wore thick glasses. He would always raise his hand to ask questions, or to give a comment, and he introduced himself as a scientist. One of the last lectures I took in was all about organic gardening, touching on GMOs. Our lecturer, a woman, filled us with emotional outrage at the use of pesticides and insecticides, and the unscrupulous practices of large-scale farming. A particularly serious note was that pesticides and insecticides were commonly carcinogenic ... promoting cancer. My scientist friend raised his hand when questions were invited, and went to great length to explain that plants usually contained their own pesticides and insecticides ... chemical compounds designed to ward off predators. He explained that these compounds were usually carcinogenic as well, and that, unlike sprayed-on man-made chemicals, could not be washed off and easily neutralized. He used green sprouts as an example, saying that plants at this particularly vulnerable stage were saturated with their own species-specific chemical pesticide and insecticide. He also reminded us that the introduction of man-made pesticides and insecticides is what made the 'green revolution' of the '60s and 70s possible, which saved our growing world population from certain famine.

The lecture ended, and a number of persons rushed toward our scientist to question him on what he had said. The first to reach him was a middle-aged woman, a vegetarian I judged, from her thinness and the dullness of her hair. "Are you saying," she questioned rather loudly, "that these plants are not good for us to eat? …. But God gave us these plants to eat!!" Our petite scientist scrutinized her through his thick lens, and replied: "I'm very sorry to be the one to tell you this, maam, *but those plants do not want you to eat them!*"

My uncontrolled snort turned several faces in my direction, and, embarrassed, yet amused, I turned and left.

The gist of the story is, of courses, that we take life regardless of our food source, whether it is animal or plant. And DNA science now tells us that the line between animal and plant life is not so distinct. This, then, is another counter argument to the vegan point of view.

The vegetarian option … vitamin B-12

The science of nutrition underscores that it is difficult to obtain all of our needed nutrients, and in sufficient quantities, if constricted to a plant-only diet. There are simply too many short-comings.

As a first example, and regardless of what you might hear a vegetarian tell you, there is no source of the essential vitamin B-12 in plants. If some B-12 is found in, say, spirulina, it is due to contamination. A true vegan diet, then, will not supply any vitamin B-12, unless supplements are taken.

The vegetarian option … protein

A vegetarian diet is usually deficient in many other nutrients as well. For example, it is not easy to obtain adequate amounts of complete proteins. A 'complete' protein is defined as a protein containing all nine essential amino acids (the ninth, histidine, however, is only essential for infants). If one of the essential amino acids is present in only a small amount in a given protein, and this 'limits' the use of the protein to make other proteins within the body, then that amino acid is termed a 'limiting' amino acid. Plants sources of protein are always lacking in one or more essential amino acids, either entirely, or having only a small amount. The grains are usually deficient in one or more of the three amino acids: lysine, threonine, or tryptophan. Legumes are mostly deficient in the sulfur-containg amino acids, methionine and cystine. Milk and dairy products are low in methionine and cystine as well, plus tryptophan and possibly lysine. The suggested solution is to 'mix' the foods, such as mixing grains and legumes, but this is not easily done, and the timing must be right … proteins are digested and especially utilized very quickly in the body. This is a point misunderstood by even many nutritionists: once a protein is digested, free amino acids in the blood are picked up by the various cells in the body very rapidly … and if the amino acids available to them do not meet those required to make the protein they are trying to make, the nitrogen head of the amino acid is quickly removed and excreted from the body as urea, and the remaining amino acid 'tail' is then sent to the Kreb Cycle for use as energy. This is why a 'complete' arsenal of amino acids must be available from the intake source at almost the same time. Although needed amino acids *can* be obtained by catabolism of existing body muscle tissue, the body treats this as a 'last resort' and does not do this quickly …it is therefore *not* true that ingesting a grain at one meal, for example, will supply the deficient amino acids in a later meal of legumes. And this is why a vegan diet will easily lead to a deficiency in useful protein. (*Advanced Nutrition and Human Metabolism,* 2005)

Current scientific consensus concludes that adults typically need a *minimum* of 0.66 grams of protein per kilogram of body weight, and the recommended adequate intake is 0.8 grams per kilogram of body weight. Therefore, for a person weighing 68 kilograms (150 pounds), the minimum requirement would be 45 grams of protein, and the recommended amount would be 54 grams. This is in keeping with the 1989 RDA recommendations. The USDA Food And Nutrition Information Center (FNIC) currently recommends the following RDAs: 9.1 grams/day for infants 0-6 months, based on 1.5 grams per kilogram weight; 11.0 grams/day for infants 6-12 months; 13 g/d for 1-3 year olds; 19g/d for 4-8 yrs; 34 g/d for male and females 9-13 yrs; 46 g/d for females 14 yrs and older; 52 g/d for males 14-18 yrs; 56 g/d for males 19 yrs and older; and 71 g/d for pregnant and lactating women of all ages.

Spokespersons from the vegetarian camp have debated that we don't need as much protein as recommended, and especially argue that high protein intakes interfere with calcium absorption and retention. Move about this further on.

The argument that we don't need as much protein as recommended is one curious part of the vegetarian logic, and perhaps deserves some clarification. I have watched this debate unfold ever since I was a teenager. It is a fascinating story. Prior to the 1970s recommended protein intakes were quite high ... the 1936 League of Nations expert committee had recommended "not less than 1 gram of protein per kilogram of body weight per day" (Scrimshaw, 2010). This would mean that an individual weighing 68 kilograms (150 pounds) would need about 68 grams of protein per day.

During the 50s and 60s it was commonly thought that we needed even more, and Adele Davis was the leading nutrition guru of the time. I remember my mother taking me to one of her lectures. She was a large woman, with black hair and masculine features, and spoke with a deep, manly voice. She was also a chain-smoker, constantly puffing on a cigarette even at the podium, and during her lectures she would be asked why she smoked so much ... she would shrug it off as a bad habit. Adele Davis was a genuine, fully accredited nutritionist, however, and the author of more than seven books on nutrition, beginning with *Optimum Health in 1939*. But she is most noted for her 4-book best-seller series *Let's Cook it Right, Let's Have Healthy Children, Let's Eat Right to Keep Fit, and Let's Get Well*, spanning the years 1947 to 1965. She argued strongly that the importance of protein could not be understated, advising intakes of 80 grams per day and even more. The general support in the science and nutrition community for high protein intake continued until 1973, when two key researchers ... the internationally renowned nutritionist, Nevin Scrimshaw, and his equally famous colleague, Vernon R. Young, who were then both working at the Massachusetts Institute of Technology ... published a landmark study which set the human requirement for protein as low as 0.34 grams per kilogram of body weight. For a 68 kilogram individual (150 pounds) this would equate to a requirement of only 23 grams of protein per day. The United Nations FAO/WHO expert committee at the time, along with most of the current scientific community, immediately accepted this new standard ... the 0.34 g/kg/d was adjusted to 0.44 g/kg/d for variability, and a maximum of 0.57 g/kg/d. Scrimshaw and Young were surprised at this almost unanimous and immediate acceptance of their study, and hastened to check their work. They had also meant this intake level to apply only to specific conditions in Guatemala, where Scrimshaw was working. They discovered that they had made a mistake in their calculations, and attempted to notify the scientific community of their error. But they were too late ... it was not until 1981 that they were finally able to re-convince WHO and the rest of the world that the range should be 0.60 – 0.75 g/kg/d. Young went on to do more work in this field, later applying a new technique using stable isotopes to measure protein balance, and became the recognized leader in this field. Just before his death in 2004 he had concluded from his work that protein requirements should be adjusted even further upwards, to 0.83 g/kg/d.

After the universal 1973 downward adjustment in recommended protein intakes the vegetarian community was quick to take advantage of the new levels, using this to illustrate that their long-asserted claim for a lower need for protein was justified. And they have not accepted the upward adjustments that took place in the 1980s and since.

The vegetarian option ... calcium

Enough calcium is also very difficult to obtain. Despite a lot of rhetoric to the contrary, it is not really plentiful in our edible plants. Following is a table showing the calcium content in selected plant foods ... the most calcium-dense source for each category. I have used data direct from the USDA Nutrient Data Base, Release 22, and have compared the calcium content to that contained in one 8-ounce glass of cow's milk, plus I have entered the amount of each food that would provide the full daily recommended amount of calcium for normal, healthy adults (RDA = 1000 mg). The USDA data conveniently lists the content amount in milligrams per 100 gram serving, plus that contained in normal measuring quantities. For vegetables, legumes, and nuts the typical quantity measure is one cup, for fruit it is the weight measure of a medium-sized fruit. The choice of cooking status was 'cooked, boiled, without salt' for the vegetables and legumes, 'dry roasted' for the nuts, and 'raw' for the fruits.

TABLE 3

Calcium Content of Selected Plant Foods

Comparison with calcium content of cow's milk

One 8 oz. cup of milk = 226 grams = 282 mg calcium

NOTE: All vegetable and legume plant foods are cooked, boiled, without salt; nuts are all dry roasted, fruits are per weight or per fruit

Food Choice	Calcium per 100 g	Calcium per cup	Amount to equal Ca content of 8 oz. milk	Amount to meet RDA of 1000 mg
Vegetables				
Soybeans	145 mg	261 mg	1.1 cups	3.8 cups
Turnip greens	137 mg	197 mg	1.4 cups	5.1 cups
Collards	140 mg	210 mg	1.3 cups	4.8 cups
Spinach	136 mg	245 mg	1.2 cups	4.1 cups
Beet greens	114 mg	164 mg	1.7 cups	6.1 cups
Okra	77 mg	62 mg	4.5 cups	16.1 cups
Mustard greens	74 mg	104 mg	2.7 cups	9.6 cups
Kale	72 mg	94 mg	3.0 cups	10.6 cups
Chard, Swiss	58 mg	102 mg	2.8 cups	9.8 cups
Cabbage	46 mg	36 mg	7.8 cups	27.8 cups
Celery	42 mg	63 mg	4.5 cups	15.9 cups
Broccoli	40 mg	31 mg	9.1 cups	32.3 cups
Parsnips	37 mg	29 mg	9.7 cups	34.5 cups
Lettuce, leaf	36 mg	13 mg	21.7 cups	76.7 cups
Brussels sprouts	36 mg	28 mg	10.1 cups	35.7 cups
Carrots	30 mg	41 mg	6.9 cups	24.4 cups
Legumes				
Peanuts	55 mg	99 mg	2.8 cups	10.1 cups
Pinto beans	46 mg	79 mg	3.6 cups	12.7 cups
Snap beans	44 mg	55 mg	5.1 cups	18.2 cups
Nuts				

82

Brazilnuts	160 mg	213 mg	1.3 cups	4.7 cups
Hazelnuts	123 mg	166 mg	1.7 cups	6.0 cups
Pistachio nuts	110 mg	135 mg	2.1 cups	7.4 cups
Pecan nuts	72 mg	97 mg	2.9 cups	10.3 cups
Walnuts	61 mg	76 mg	3.7 cups	13.2 cups
Butternuts	53 mg	64 mg	4.4 cups	15.6 cups
Fruits				
Raisins	53 mg	77 mg	3.6 cups	13.0 cups
Oranges	40 mg	52 mg / fruit	5.4 oranges	19.2 oranges
Dates	39 mg	57 mg	4.9 cups	17.5 cups
Elderberries	38 mg	55 mg	5.1 cups	18.2 cups
Kiwi fruit	34 mg	23 mg / fruit	12.3 fruit	43.5 fruit
Jackfruit	34 mg	56 mg	5.0 cups	17.9 cups
Grains				
Granola	78 mg	95 mg	2.9 cups	10.5 cups
Oat flour	55 mg	74 mg	3.8 cups	13.5 cups
Oats	54 mg	84 mg	3.4 cups	11.9 cups
Buckwheat flour	41 mg	49 mg	5.8 cups	20.4 cups
Wheat flour	34 mg	41 mg	6.9 cups	24.4 cups
Barley flour	32 mg	47 mg	6.0 cups	21.3 cups
Spirulina	120 mg	134 mg	2.1 cups	7.5 cups

In addition, fibers, phytates, oxalate, and competition from other divalent minerals often interferes with bioavailability. This is particulary the case with many of our green-leaf plant foods. Non-digestible fibers such as cellulose or those found in wheat bran can increase the bulk of intestinal contents and cause the food mass to move rapidly through the small intestine, thereby decreasing transit time, and lessening the time available for calcium absorption. Phytate in legumes, nuts, and cereals can bind with calcium and prevent its absorption as well. The presence of oxalate may also be an inhibiting factor for absorption. The oxalate chelates the calcium (forms a closed molecular or atom chain) and prevents digestion in the small intestine, causing the compound to be excreted as part of fecal matter. Oxalate is found in a number of vegetables, such as spinach, beets, celery, eggplant, greens, okra, and squash; or in fruits such as strawberries, blackberries, blueberries, gooseberries, and currants; in nuts such as pecans and peanuts; and in beverages such as tea, Ovaltine, and cocoa. The calcium ion has a double positive charge, or is divalent. So is zinc, the ferric form of iron, and magnesium. Magnesium is known to especially compete with calcium for intestinal absorption, particularly when there is an excess of one or the other. A vegan diet can thus seriously limit the availability of bioavailable calcium.

The vegetarian option ... iron

Iron is another problem, and iron deficiency is much more common among vegetarians. This is largely because iron in plants (*non-heme iron*) is much less bioavailable than iron found in animal foods (*heme iron*). Heme iron, which is part of a pre-formed *porphyrin ring* is readily absorbed intact into the muscal cell of the small intestine. Nonheme iron, however, is normally bound to components of plant foods and must be liberated in the gastrointestinal tract prior to absorption. This liberation process frees the iron ions in either the ferrous form (having a positive charge of 3), or as ferric iron (having a positive charge of 2), depending on conditions in the stomach and small intestine ... but only the ferrous form is soluble and can pass through the intestinal membranes into the blood stream. The ferric form will tend to be insoluble and is also more easily chelated ... both events tending to cause the iron to be unabsorbed and excreted as part of fecal matter, similarly to non-absorbed calcium. (*Advanced Nutrition and Human Metabolism, 2005*).

These nutrient problems with the vegan diet tend to result in lower growth rates and decreased stature. When you hear the defensive statement, "small but healthy", consider it to be total nonsense ... stunting, or below-normal stature, is an almost universal indicator of poor nutrition status. A person on a vegan diet will frequently have low body strength, and low stamina. In addition, a vegan will often have dull, lifeless hair, due to the lack of protein. And, in my own experience, their temperament is noticeably fragile ... only my own biased observation, of course.

My own careful opinion is that the vegetarian option is the *ideal* ... it is a very worthwhile goal ... but it must be approached with knowledge and planning ... and our plant food supply base needs to be greatly improved.

6. Animal rights sentiments

When it comes to the issue of eating the flesh and flesh-products of other animals for food, I am reminded of a poignant scene in the recent version of *War of the Worlds*, starring no less than our super hero, Tom Cruise. The new version has a couple of twists from the original, which I remember haunted me in my youth. The aliens, it is revealed, used earth as a 'farm' for growing edible humans, and had planted machines in the earth at some distant time in the past, in anticipation of 'harvest time'. The scene that is stuck so vividly in my mind is that of the monster machines stalking helpless humans running frantically beneath them, sapping them with a sort of lazer gun, followed by a long hose-like appendix shooting out, stabbing the helpless and not yet dead human victim, sucking the body dry of blood ... the corpse twitching and flapping in auto-reflex spasms. It flashed on me, being thoroughly stunned by the full impact of this gruesome scene, that this is not very far removed from how we humans treat our domesticated food animals.

As a youngster I remember one Christmas family reunion when Uncle Irvin and his helpers corralled a frantically squealing pig and strung him high by the hind legs. The first move was to thrust a long-bladed knife into its neck and up towards its heart, and Auntie stood by with a small pail to catch its blood ... to make a delicious blood pie, I was told. Then the animal was butchered and dissected ... to become the main course for our grand feast to follow. I was five at the time, and the scene deeply disturbed me.

Or, a scene from *The Texas Chain-Saw Massacre*, showing cattle docilely riding a mechanized conveyor-ramp, rising up to the entrance of a large barn-looking building, where a husky red-necked executioner waited with his sledge hammer, delivering a single and precise blow to the animal's forehead at the correct moment. The ensuing butchering process then proceeded unemotionally, the animal carcasses suspended on an overhead, downward sloping rail system, the weight of the corpses motorizing the system.

Are we, then, any different from those horrible aliens, hunting down Tom Cruise and his fellow citizens for their blood?

Now, you might argue that taking the milk from the udder of a well-cared for cow is not the same thing. Or is it?

7. <u>Trends in the dairy industry ... big business</u>

Although dairy farms in America are still predominately family-owned operations, with the over-all national average of the number of cows per farm only 120, the trend is in the direction of mega-sized dairies, with the state of California taking the lead. It is a familiar story ... small, family operated businesses going under, big business moving in and monopolizing the sector. Between 1970 and 2006 the number of farms with dairy cows fell from 648,000 to 105,000. The number of dairy cows fell from 12 million to 9.1 million, and the average herd size rose from 19 to 120. However, because milk production per cow more than doubled, from 9,751 to 19,951 pounds per year, total milk production increased ... with the average milk production per farm increasing 12-fold. Milk production from farms having more than 500 milking cows in California accounts for 88% of total state production, which in turn accounted for 21% of national output in 2006. On a national level, the number of dairy farms with a dairy herd size greater than 2,000 grew from 280 in 2000 to 573 in 2006 (USDA). During the same period, farms with less than 100 cows fell from 84,220 to 57,640.

Spokespersons for the dairy industry argue that there is essentially no difference between how milking cows are treated in larger sized dairies compared to smaller, more family orientated operations. However, observational evidence says different. The major negative differences between large-scale dairies and small ones can be summarized as follows:

1. Small farms tend to keep their dairy herd outside, allowing them to roam and feed in pastures ... larger enterprises tend to keep the animals housed inside, feeding them grains instead of pasture grasses, and not allowing the animals to roam open pasture.

2. Dairy farms with smaller herds dispose of their manure waste by allowing it to be naturally spread in pasture land, while the big operations must resort to the construction of large 'manure ponds'.

3. Larger dairies are more likely to practice the injection of their dairy herd with 'recombinant bovine growth hormone' (rBGH) to increase milk production ... there has been a growing resistance by smaller dairy operators to use rBGH.

The most common grain feeds for dairy cattle are corn and soybean. Statistics for use of pesticides on plant crops in the U.S. indicate that 70% of total pesticide use is on fields of corn and soybeans, of which 67% are used for feed for dairy cattle. Although these feeds are superior to natural pasture grasses in some respects, they are not the animal's natural food and are not fully compatible with a cow's digestive system. . It is known that corn and soy cause health problems in the cow, requiring increased use of anti-biotics. So, not only are housed dairy cows ingesting more pesticides through the corn and soy, they are given additional antibiotics to combat the infections caused by the feed.

Measured by the phosphorus content, the waste output of 5,000 cows roughly equals a town of 70,000 people. In a normal small farm operation, manure is utilized for cropland fertilization or is disposed of in the field, at the ratio of about 5 or 6 cows to the acre. Mega farms instead construct large manure ponds and methane digesters, which can cover several acres in area. On August 10th, 2005, a giant manure lagoon collapsed at a 5,000-cow dairy in upstate New York, releasing several million gallons of manure into the Black River. It was estimated that 375,000 fish were killed, plus creating a major pollution disaster. The New York Department of Environmental Conservation fined the dairy $2.2 million.

One example of the role of big business in the dairy industry is the story of recombinant bovine growth hormone (rBGH) and the massive corporation, Monsanto. This story is unfolded later in this chapter, but it is important to note here that the administration of rBGH is used in the U.S. to increase milk production, but is banned in the EU, Canada, Australia, New Zealand, and Japan because of evidence of resulting harm to both the cow and humans. As mentioned elsewhere in this chapter, a USDA survey in 2007 estimated that rBGH was being administered to 17.2% of all U.S. dairy cows. Because milk is mixed during commercial preparation and distribution, and also in the making of other dairy products, such as yogurt and cheeses, it is likely that a large portion of the milk consumed by Americans contains some amount of rBGH milk.

Insights to modern dairy industry practices

The historical process of innovations and changing dairy-farm practices illustrates the trend toward increased mechanization and larger dairies. The transition from the traditional milking pail to the ultra-modern vacuum and piping systems of today is an intriguing study.

One early improvement was the installation of a simple milker device that fit on top of the milking pail. This then developed into the 'Surge' hanging milker, which incorporated a large wide leather strap called a 'surcingle' placed around the cow, across the cow's lower back. The milker device and collection tank hung from the strap underneath the cow. This innovation allowed the cow to move around during the milking process, rather than having to stand perfectly still over a bucket placed on the floor.

With the availability of electric power and the invention of suction milking machines, the production levels that were possible in stanchion barns increased further, but the scale of the operations continued to be limited by the labor intensive nature of the milking process ... the milker was still required to carry the milk pail to the storage tank. The next innovation was then a vacuum milk-transport system known as the Step-Saver, which transported milk from the cow to the storage tank. Next came the milk pipeline, using a permanent milk-return pipe and a second vacuum pipe that encircled the barn or milking parlor above the rows of cows, with quick-seal entry ports above each cow. By thus eliminating the need for the milk container, the milking device was reduced in size and weight to the point where it could hang under the cow, held up only by the sucking force of the milker nipples on the cow's udder. In this system the milk is pulled up into the milk-return pipe by the vacuum system, and then flows by gravity to the storage tank.

The next major step towards increased automation and assembly-line systems was the introduction of 'milking parlors'. The basic concept behind the milking parlor was to maximize the number of cows that a single operator could handle. Physical stress on the farmer is reduced by positioning the cows on a platform slightly above the person milking the cows, eliminating the need for the milker to bend over. The milking parlor allowed a concentration of money into a small area, so that more technical monitoring and measuring equipment could be devoted to each milking station in the parlor. Rather than simply milking into a common pipeline for example, the parlor can be equipped with fixed measurement systems that monitor milk volume and record milking statistics for each animal. Tags on the animals allow the parlor system to automatically identify each animal as it enters the parlor. Even more modern farms use recessed parlors, where the milker stands in a recess such that his arms are at the level of the cow's udder. Recessed parlors can be herringbone, where the cows stand in two angled rows either side of the recess and the milker accesses the udder from the side, or parallel, where the cows stand side-by-side and the milker accesses the udder from the rear, or, more recently, a rotary (or carousel) configuration, where the cows are on a raised circular platform, facing the center of the circle, and the platform rotates while the milker stands in one place and accesses the udder from the rear.

In herringbone and parallel parlors, the milker generally milks one row at a time. The milker will move a row of cows from the holding yard into the milking parlor, and milk each cow in that row. Once all or most of the milking machines have been removed from the milked row, the milker releases the cows to their feed. A new group of cows is then loaded into the now vacant side and the process repeats until all cows are milked. Depending on the size of the milking parlor, which normally is the bottleneck, these rows of cows can range from four to sixty at a time.

Finally, in the 1980s and 1990s, robotic milking systems were developed and introduced, but have been used principally in the EU.

Because it can be harmful to an animal to be over-milked past the point where the udder has stopped releasing milk, the amount being removed from the cow's udder needs to be monitored. Automatic monitoring devices have therefore been developed to let the milker know when the milker should be removed, and/or an automatic take-off system removes the milker from the cow when the milk reaches a preset level.

It takes the average cow three to five minutes to give her milk. Some cows are faster than others. Slower-milking cows can take up to fifteen minutes to let down all their milk. Because milking speed is a separate factor from milk quantity, and most milkers milk the cows in groups, the milker can only process a group of cows at the speed of the slowest-milking cow. For this reason, many farmers will cull slow-milking cows.

The extracted milk passes through a strainer and plate heat exchangers before entering the tank, where it can be stored safely for a few days at approximately 42 degrees Fahrenheit (6 degrees centigrade). At a pre-arranged time, a milk truck arrives and pumps the milk from the tank for transport to a dairy factory where it will be pasteurized and processed into multiple products.

Under modern conditions, cows are usually milked two to three times a day.

The production of milk requires that the cow be in lactation, which is a result of the cow having given birth to a calf. The cycle includes insemination, pregnancy, parturition, and lactation, followed by a "dry" period of a few weeks before calving which allows udder tissue to regenerate. Insemination can be accomplished naturally by keeping a bull on hand, but this is rarely done nowadays ... instead a veterinarian artificially impregnates the cow by manually inserting a semen capsule deep into the cow's vagina. Dairy operations therefore include both the production of milk and the production of calves. Bull calves are either butchered for veal or castrated and raised as steers for beef production. Female calves become future dairy cows.

Calves born to dairy cows, the primary purpose of which is to induce lactation, are taken away either immediately after birth or within a day or so. This separation can cause great distress to the mother, who would normally feed the calf more than a dozen times a day and, like other mammals, forms a strong bond with her young soon after birth. Immediate separation is therefore necessary to reduce stress in the mother cow.

A cow's natural life expectancy is about 20 years, but the average dairy cow lives just 4 to 5 years, exhausted by constant lactation, births, and disease.

Common ailments affecting dairy cows include infectious disease (e.g. mastitis, endometritis and digital demantitis), metabolic disease (e.g. milk fever and ketosis) and injuries caused by their environment (e.g. hoof and hock lesions). Lameness is commonly considered one of the most significant animal welfare issues for dairy cattle. It can be caused by a number of sources, including infections of the hoof tissue (e.g. fungal infections that cause dermatitis) and physical damage causing bruising or lesions (e.g. ulcers or hemorrhage of the hoof). Housing and management features common in modern conventional dairy farms, such as concrete barn floors, limited access to pasture, and suboptimal bed-stall design have been identified as contributing risk factors.

Big business … reason for concern

The world's largest exporter of dairy products is New Zealand, where dairy products also account for the largest share of the nation's export earnings. Fonterra is New Zealand's largest company, and the fifth-largest dairy company in the world. More about Fonterra in the next chapter.

U.S. milk prices collapsed in 2009, and big business was blamed. Senator Bernie Sanders accused Dean Foods of price manipulation, citing the statistic that the company controls 40% of the country's milk market. He has requested the United States Department of Justice to pursue 'an anti-trust investigation". Dean Foods counters that it buys only 15% of the country's raw milk.

Currently, concerns regarding monopolies created by Dean Foods, Kraft, and other major buyers of bulk dairy products have been raised, as American dairy farms have suffered extreme price depression and chaotic fluctuations while processors and retailers report record profits. Many theorize, for example, that unregulated imports of milk protein concentrate used by processors to boost cheese yield has artificially and unfairly influenced the markets in an effort to force consolidation and vertical integration in what has historically been a highly diversified industry ... in other words, big business is manipulating in order to control the market. (Wikipedia)

Nocton Dairies

Until very recently the trend towards domination of the dairy industry by big business has been mostly an American phenomenon ... but it is now spreading to other countries. Nocton Dairies, for example, had planned the construction of the first mega-sized dairy outside the U.S., to begin construction in 2010 in Nocton Heath, Lincolnshire, England. The facility would have housed 8,100 dairy cows, and promised to produce "high-welfare, low carbon" milk. However, pressure from animal rights groups, led by 'Compassion in World Farming' succeeded in blocking Nocton's construction application. On April 15, 2010, 172 Members of Parliament voted against the application. The primary issue presented by the various animal welfare organizations was the dairy's plans to keep the cows inside and feed them cereals, rather than allow them free access to pasture. Nevertheless, Nocton has announced plans to advance with a second planning application. (AFN, 2010)

Movies and documentaries ... our food supply and big business

The 2006 movie *Fast Food Nation* was a recent attempt to dramatize and bring attention to the sometimes dubious and unethical management of our food supply by big business. The script was written by Richard Linklater and the investigative reporter, Eric Schlosser, and was based on Schlosser's 2001 bestselling non-fiction book of the same name. The movie was designed as a drama rather than a documentary, but was essentially a parody of McDonald's and Burger King's big business fast-food outlets and style of organization. Although the reviews did not give the movie a very high scoring, it did succeed in drawing attention to the sometimes unscrupulous maneuvering of big business in the fast-food business, and won 6 awards and nominations.

Eric Schlosser again plays an important role in another movie/documentary which was unveiled this past summer (2010), entitled *Food, Inc.* Filmmaker Robert Kenner reveals that our American food supply is controlled by a handful of corporations that often place profit ahead of the health of consumers, the welfare of the farmer, the safety of workers, the care of the environment, and the well-being of the animals we raise for food. The documentary features interviews with Eric Schlosser, Michael Pollan (*The Omnivore's Dilemna, In Defense of food: An Eater's Manifesto)*, Gary Hirshberg (Stoneyfield Organic Farms), and Joel Salatin (Polyface Farms). Exposed is the highly mechanized underbelly of the American food industry and the story about what we eat, how it's produced, and the affect on our individual and national health status.

8. rBGH, Monsanto, IGF-1, and more

As early as 1937 it was known that the hormone *bovine somatotropin* (BST) could be taken from bovine cadavers and administered to live cows to increase their milk yield. The yield increase was as high as 25 percent. Another name for this same hormone is *bovine growth hormone*, or BGH. During the 1980s four separate American chemical/pharmaceutical companies carried out extensive research with the goal of creating an artificial or *recombinant* form of this same hormone. These companies were Upjohn, Eli Lily, American Cyanamid, and Monsanto. Collectively, these companies invested over $1 billion in research and development. Applying the-then-new recombinant DNA technology, Monsanto scientists were the first to succeed ... they genetically modify a plant cell in 1982, and later were able to genetically modify an *E. coli* cell by inserting the gene that codes the sequence of amino acids that make up BST, and then process the bacteria further to produce the injectable hormone. The new product was named *Prosilac*.

Instructions for the injection of Posilac recommended that the injection be made about 50 days into the cow's natural lactation period, just before the animal peaked its milk production ... the Posilac then causes the high rate of production to continue, and later to decline more slowly than normal.

Prosilac was approved for sale by the FDA November 5, 1993, with the provision that a 90-day moratorium be placed on actual sales. The moratorium expired on February 3, 1994, and Prosilac went on sale the next day.

When I began researching the rBGH and Monsanto story, I was deeply troubled to read about Monsanto's long history of producing potentially harmful chemical products, genetically modified crop seeds, and with a parallel history of legal entanglement in all sorts of lawsuits, both as defendant and plaintiff. The Monsanto story reads like a movie-script of a ruthless and immoral corporation giant savagely extorting profit in any way it can, totally unmindful of environmental and human sensitivities, seemingly bent only on the accumulation of power and wealth. Its reported gross revenue for 2008 was $11.365 billion USD, with a net income of $2.024 billion.

The questionable chemicals produced over the years by Monsanto include the herbicides DDT and 2,4,5-T, plus the toxic chemicals used in transformers, known collectively as 'PCBs', and the defoliant Agent Orange used by the American forces in the Vietnam War. Dioxin residues and contamination have been a frequent issue.

Monsanto was sued in the longest civil jury trial in U.S. history by a group of plaintiffs who claimed they were poisoned by dioxin in a 1979 chemical spill that occurred in Sturgeon, Missouri. Monsanto won.

In August of 2003 Monsanto and one of their spin-off companies, Solutia, agreed to pay $700 million to over 20,000 residents of Anniston, Alabama in restitution for having unlawfully and without regard to the environment nor residents, discharged both mercury and PCB-laden waste into local creeks over a period of 40 years. Monsanto had also buried millions of pounds of PCB in open-pit landfills located on hillsides above the plant and surrounding neighborhoods.

Monsanto has been identified by the U.S. Environmental Protection Agency as being a "potentially responsible party" for 56 major contamination sites in the U.S.

Agent Orange was a 50:50 mix of 2,4-D and 2,4,5-T herbicides, and was manufactured by 37 different companies, with the largest shares produced by Dow Chemical and Monsanto. The herbicide was known to be toxic, especially if contaminated by the dioxin 2,3,7,8-tetrachlordibenzo-para-dioxin (TCDD). The levels of TCDD in the domestic version of the Monsanto herbicide during the time was about 0.05 parts-per-million … that shipped to Vietnam peaked at 50 ppm … a 1,000 times higher concentration. It was for this reason that the presiding judge in the 1984 out-of-court settlement to 291,000 American GIs required that Monsanto pay 45.5% of the $180 million settlement.

But Monsanto has successfully won against any further legal suits for its role in the Agent Orange saga, including further suits by American GIs and the Vietnamese themselves. Yet, the saga is not over ... Monsanto is still under fire for inconsistencies in its own studies and defense, including the cover-up of information that indicated that the company was well aware of the dangers of dioxins to humans as far back as 1949.

In 2009 the Department of Veterans Affairs added three more 'presumed' illnesses associated with Agent Orange exposure. Damage benefits from exposure to Agent Orange can now be claimed by veterans for a total of 15 disease conditions, which are: B cell leukemia, Parkinson's Disease, ischemic heart diseases, acute and subacute transient peripheral neuropathy, cloracne, chronic lymphocytic leukemia, type 2 diabetes mellitus, Hodgkin's Disease, multiple myeloma, non-Hodgkin's lymphoma, porphyria cutanea tarda, prostate cancer, respiratory cancers, and soft tissue sarcoma (other than osteosarcoma, chondrosarcoma, Kaposi's Sarcoma, or mesothelioma). (Young, 2009)

During the 1980s Monsanto re-aligned their product strategy and entered the newly emerging field of agricultural biotechnology, producing a variety of genetically modified crop seeds. Their technology and marketing strategy was both innovative and unique. They first modified their seeds to be resistant to their top selling and very successful herbicide, *Roundup*. Roundup is a strong defoliant, able to kill all weeds and other vegetation with a single application ... their advertising cliché is 'one shot does it all'. The concept is that their seed is planted, and then the field of young crop plants is sprayed with Roundup, thereby killing all vegetation, yet leaving the main crop plant unharmed. The technique is very effective. However, each purchaser of the Monsanto Roundup-resistant seed is required, in writing, to honor Monsanto's patent and property rights, which includes barring the saving of a portion of one crops seed for subsequent plantings ... new seed must be purchased for each new planting. And of course the farmer is required to purchase the Roundup herbicide.

This strategy seems reasonable enough, except that Monsanto has used this technique and marketing scheme to control the seed market and to force a growing percentage of farmers to use their seed and herbicide. They first of all aggressively bought up almost all of the other seed manufacturers on a world-wide scale and then went after farmers who were saving seeds or who had genetically modified plants in their fields, even without knowing it. Taking advantage of the common observation that plant seeds can travel long distances to contaminate or mix with plant seeds in another area, Monsanto has investigated fields of unsuspecting farmers and then sued them for illegally growing their GM crops. A recent estimate is that Monsanto has collected more than $200 million from farmers thus far via this ruthless strategy. In addition, through massive and questionable lobbying tactics and considerable expense, Monsanto was able to prevent legislation in the U.S. that would allow producers to label agricultural products as free from genetic modification (GM).

Monsanto spent $8,831,120 for lobbying in the year 2008, of which $1,492,000 was to outside lobbying firms ... the remainder for in-house lobbying expenses. (Wikipedia, 2010)

Neil Hart, agricultural economist at Iowa State University and an authority on the seed industry, states: "We now believe that Monsanto has control over as much as 90 percent of seed genetics. This level of control is almost unbelievable." (.docstoc)

The end effect is that Monsanto monopolizes not only the seed market, but crop technology and farming practices as well. As one farmer, sued by Monsanto for allegedly saving seed for re-planting, suggests, "They are in the process of owning food, all food." Another adds, "Its objective is to control all of the world's food production." Vandan Shiva, well-known Indian physicist and activist, puts it even more poignantly: "If they control seed, they control food; they know it, it's strategic. It's more powerful than bombs; it's more powerful than guns. This is the best way to control the population of the world."

Two Monsanto policy statements and a court ruling are indicative of their position on the way they do business. In 1998 Monsanto's Director of Corporate Communications, in reference to the U.S. Food and Drug Administration, stated: "Monsanto should not have to vouchsafe the safety of biotech food. Our interest is in selling as much as possible. Assuring its safety is FDA's job." A Monsanto memo explaining their justification for hiding the truth about 40 years of pollution from Anniston, Alabama residents proclaimed: "We can't afford to lose one dollar of business."

In the Anniston case Monsanto was convicted of negligence, wantonness, suppression of the truth, nuisance, trespass, and *outrage*. According to Alabama law, to be guilty of 'outrage' requires conduct "so outrageous in character and extreme in degree as to go beyond all possible bounds of decency so as to be regarded as atrocious and utterly intolerable in civilized society." (Grunwald, 2002)

However, Monsanto is now facing a new threat to their marketing strategy and dominance ... *the invasion of the superweeds* !! The seemingly inevitable has happened ... new Roundup-resistant varieties of plants have been showing up across the country. William Neuman and Andrew Pollack write that "The first resistant species to a pose a serious threat to agriculture was spotted in a Delaware soybean field in 2000. Since then, the problem has spread, with 10 resistant species in at least 22 states infesting millions of acres, predominantly soybeans, cotton and corn." Andrew Wargo III, president of the Arkansas Association of Conservation Districts, states "It is the single largest threat to production agriculture that we have ever seen." (PPJ Gazette, May 6, 2010)

Back to rBGH

A search in the library, on the internet, and in Medline, surfaced no studies to show that rBGH is harmful to humans. But that is not the end of it. A review of how rBGH came to be developed, how it became approved by the FDA, and the broad view of how it can affect both cow's and humans, reveals several disturbing findings. First, it is now known that rBGH injected into the dairy cow can result in a series of unhealthy consequences for the animal, often requiring further treatment with anti-biotics, residues of which can be passed on to humans through the milk. Secondly, administrations of rBGH in cows significantly increases the level of IGF-1 in the animal and is passed to its milk ... IGF-1 has been shown to have links with several disease conditions in humans. Thirdly, Monsanto originally argued successfully with the FDA that the IGF-1 found in the milk of cow's treated with rBGH is destroyed by pasteurization and/or by acids in the human stomach ... it is now known that this argument was based on bad science and misconception. Further studies have indicated that IGF-1 can survive pasteurization and stomach acids, and can pass through intestinal walls, and can then contribute to disease conditions in humans.

rBGH and animal health

Two much-referenced mega studies conducted by Dohoo et al find that with "an average increase in milk output ranging from 11 – 16%, (resulted in) a nearly 25% increase in the risk of clinical mastitis (inflammation of the udder), a 40% reduction in fertility and 55% increased risk of developing clinical signs of lameness." (Dohoo, 2003)

rBGH and IGF-1

The 'insulin-like growth factor-1' (IGF-1) in dairy cows is identical to the same hormone in humans. IGF-1 is also named 'somatomedin C'. The compound is a polypeptide (a protein) produced mainly in the liver, in response to the growth hormone (GH) which is released from the pituitary gland. The growth hormone then stimulates the liver to excrete IGF-1, which in turn acts on a large number of different body tissues to enhance growth. One role is to stimulate cell division and cell differentiation ... and is therefore 'mitogenic' ... and can potentially play a role in the formation of various cancers. The level of IGF-1 is known to increase when a cancer condition is evidenced, especially with prostate and breast cancer.

The consensus in the scientific community currently supports findings that (a) rBGH administration to dairy cows increases the level of IGF-1 in their milk, that (b) this additional IGF-1 *is* absorbed by humans, and that (c) the result is an increase in the human level of IGF-1. This consensus has taken a long time to emerge, largely because the FDA and other scientists had originally accepted Monsanto's claims that first showed no increase in IGF-1 in rBGH- treated cow's, and then that the IGF-1 was destroyed by pasteurization or could not survive the acid conditions of the human digestion environment. It was finally concluded that Monsanto's studies and conclusions were flawed.

The current debate, however, is whether a high level of IGF-1 is an indicator of the disease condition, and perhaps even a mediator, or if it plays a causal role in the initiation and progress of disease conditions. Jane Plant, in her 1988 book, *Your Life In Your Hands: Understanding, Preventing And Overcoming Breast Cancer*, (Plant, 1988), submits evidence and scientific studies available at that time that IGF-1 is directly linked to breast cancer. Robert Cohen, author of *Milk, The Deadly Poison* (Cohen, 1998), and sponsor of the website www.notmilk.com , adds to Plant's list of studies and concludes that IGF-1 plays a causal role in prostate and colon cancer as well. Another book presenting similar findings is *The Milk Imperative,* by Russel Eaton (Eaton, 2006). Numerous research articles have been published as well ... I list a few of these in the reference and comment section for this chapter, with each article's conclusion.

It is interesting that artificial IGF-1 steroids have been available for some years now for body-building enthusiasts. Many body-builders claim that the injection of IGF-1 into specific muscle sites enhances the growth of that muscle tissue. Fitness literature cites advantages such as increased muscle cell growth, heightened protein anabolism, improved protein balance, and assisted amino acid shuttling into muscles. Noted side effects include nausea, hypoglycemia (low blood sugar), headaches, dizziness, and accelerated growth of existing cancerous tumors. The body-building experience tends to support the potential for IGF-1 to promote both cancer and diabetes.

Banned in Canada, the European Union, Australia, New Zealand, and Japan.

The European Union had already placed a moratorium on genetically modified foods in 1990, even before Monsanto had obtained FDA approval in the U.S. (1994). Health Canada issued a formal "notice of non-compliance" in January, 1999, disapproving of any future sales of rBGH and its use with dairy cows. The position was based on the conclusions by the expert committees on veterinary and human safety under the auspicies of the Canadian Veterinary Medical Association and the Royal College of Physicians and Surgeons, which in particular noted an increase in the incidence of mastitis, lameness, and reproductive problems among treated dairy cows. Two expert committees commissioned by the European Union in the same year confirmed the Canadian conclusions and also supported findings that rBGH milk contained higher levels of Insulin-like-Growth Factor One (IGF-1) and concluded that this posed a major risk for cancer, particularly breast and prostate cancers. A permanent ban on the sale and use of rBGH was adopted by all 25 EU member nations in January, 2000. New Zealand, Australia, and Japan followed suit shortly thereafter. These bans remain in effect as of this writing.

Codex Alimentiarius, the U.N. Food Safety Agency, as a conclusion to their 23rd Session (1999), officially agreed to shelve any further discussion of a U.S.-backed proposal to set a Maximum Residue Level (MRL) for rBGH. By indefinitely shelving the proposal, Codex acknowledged the deep division between countries such as the U.S., that insist rBGH is safe and countries like those of the European Union, where rBGH has not been approved due to nagging safety concerns. (Linger, 1999)

The revolving door scenario … and Monsanto

In a functional democracy confidence in government and particularly government regulation is a key issue. Confidence is compromised whenever the independence of those making decisions, notably those empowered to regulate, is called into question. Transfers of key personnel between the 'private sector' and 'government' are particularly suspect, despite the existence of ethics laws, codes, and regulations. The Edmonds Institute has created a database which keeps track of such key players.

One example is the case of Margaret Miller and Michael Taylor. Margaret Miller was a former chemical laboratory supervisor for Monsanto, and is now Deputy Director of Human Food Safety and Consultative Services, New Animal Drug Evaluation Office, Center for Veterinary Medicine in the U.S. FDA. Michael Taylor worked as a staff lawyer for the USDA from 1976 – 81, then left government to work at King & Spaulding, a law firm representing Monsanto. In 1991 he returned to work for the U.S. government, this time for the FDA, graduating to the post of Administrator for the USDA's Food Safety & Inspection Service in 1994. His appointment had been sanctioned by then President Bill Clinton. In the same year, he and Margaret Miller, along with Suzanne Sechen (an FDA "primary reviewer for all rBGH and other dairy drug production applicatons"), were targeted by the U.S. General Accounting Office (GAO) in their investigation of their role in FDA's approval of Monsanto's Posilac.

While with the FDA, Taylor played a central role in the creation of the "substantial equivalence" concept, and the doctrine based on this principle that became almost universally accepted internationally. The concept argues that there is no difference between foods that are genetically modified and their non-GM equivalents. This became the basis for not requiring special testing or special labeling. More about this in the section on labeling.

Beginning in 2000, Taylor served as Research Professor of Health Policy at George Washington University. In July, 2009, President Obama appointed Taylor to be the senior adviser to the U.S. FDA. (Spin Profiles, 2010)

Hillary Clinton, former first lady and now Secretary of State, has connections with Monsanto going back to when she worked for the Rose Law Firm, whose prime clients were Monsanto, Tyson, and Walmart. These companies were strong backers of the Clinton administration. They stand out as leading players in genetic engineering and industrialized food. Soon after taking office, Obama appointed Tom Vilsak as head of the USDA. The appointment was opposed by 20,000 emails objecting to Vilsak's close connections with Monsanto. (OEN, 2010)

On February 22, 2010, a group of 98 separate organizations combined to present a letter to the U.S. senate opposing the appointment of Islam Siddiqui as Chief Agricultural Negotiator, Office of the United State Trade Representative. Paragraph two of the letter contains the following explanation:

"Siddigui's record at the U.S. Department of Agriculture and his role as a former registered lobbyist for CropLife America (whose members include Monsanto, Syngenta, DuPont and Dow), has revealed him to consistently favor agribusinesses' interests over the interests of consumers, the environment and public health. We believe Siddiqui's nomination severely weakens the Obama Administration's credibility in promoting healthier and more sustainable local food systems here at home. His appointment would also send an unfortunate signal to the rest of the world that the United States plans to continue down the failed path of high-input and energy-intensive industrial agriculture by promoting toxic pesticides, inappropriate seed biotechnologies and unfair trade agreements on nations that do not want and can least afford them." (Organic Consumers Association, 2010)

Siddiqui's appointment was confirmed by the US senate on March 29, 2010.

rBGH production sold to Eli Lilly

The rBGH production part of Monsanto was sold, in full, to Eli Lilly for $300 million, plus additional considerations, in October, 2008. (Wikipedia)

Due to successful Monsanto lobbying, it is still against the law to advertise milk to be free of rBGH in some American states ... the controversy and legislation in both directions is on-going. There has, however, been a growing list of producers and retailers refusing to produce or sell milk produced with rBGH. These include the nation's largest dairy processor, Dean Foods, plus Safeway (north-western states only), Walmart, Kroger, Starbucks, and Costco.

A USDA survey in 2007 estimated that rBGH was being administered to 17.2% of all U.S. dairy cows. Because milk is mixed during commercial preparation and distribution, and also in the making of other dairy products, such as yogurt and cheeses, it is likely that most of the milk consumed by Americans contains some portion of rBGH milk.

References for the rBGH controversy

A great deal has been written by various authors about the use of rBGH, mostly written with strong arguments against. One noted writer is Robert Cohen, author of *MILK, The Deadly Poison,* 1998. Cohen is a very active opponent of the use of rBGH, and has a website at www.nomilk.com. In his book Cohen leads the reader through a detailed analysis of Monsanto's research and writings, and has extensively researched each step, including tracing Monsanto's connection with the FDA and the inter-change of scientists, lawyers, and executives on their respective employee lists.. More recently is *What's In Your Milk, An Expose' of Industry and Government Cover-Up on the DANGERS of the Genetically Engineered (rBGH) Milk You're Drinking,* 2006, compiled by Dr. Samuel S. Epstein, M.D. In the reference section at the end of this chapter I have listed a number of research articles and periodical publications on the subject.

9. <u>Other things in milk ... blood, pus, manure, and toxins</u>

Yes ... there is blood and pus and manure in the cow's milk you buy at the local supermarket !!

During my late teens I worked during two summers on two separate dairy farms. It was hard work ... and I had my full share of chasing after dumb cows in the mud, shoveling manure and cleaning out barns, getting kicked for being in the wrong place at the wrong time, and struggling with bales of hay on a tractor-drawn trailer behind a baler. The two families I worked for were wonderful people ... hard-working, honest, and so very down-to-earth. When it came to taking care of their cows and producing the best milk under the best of conditions, they were unexcelled. It was while working on those two farms that I ate the best food of my life. And, of course, we drank oodles of our own milk.

Milk is screened at the farm, which removes almost all of the visible foreign matter which accidently contaminates the output, and which *does* include manure, maybe some dirt off the ground, and even a little hay or feed. I say 'almost all' is screened, because not a full 100% is removed via the simple screening process ... there is always a little that still ends up in the milk.

Cow's blood in the milk is another problem, but is visible, and any milk containing blood is quickly discarded at the farm. Very, very little ever makes it to the milk finally sent to the dairy.

Somatic cell count

The main concern of milk producers is not the minute amount of foreign matter that might accidently find its way into the farmers bulk tanks or the trucks, or the huge processing tanks at the dairy, but instead is the amount of 'somatic cells' found present in the final product. A small number of these cells can be bacteria cells, but 95% are leucocytes, which includes neutrophils, macrophages, and lymphocytes. These are, essentially, dead white blood cells ... the same cells that make up what we commonly call 'pus'. The somatic cell count (SCC), or the number of somatic cells per milliliter of milk is tested for and is highly regulated. The SCC is *not* used as a measure of contamination, however, but is used as an indicator of mammary health in the dairy cow ... it is an indicator of the animals immune response and thus the presence of infection in the udder, or mastitis. Studies on the relationship between the somatic cell count and mammary infection have slightly varying conclusions, but there is a consensus that 250,000 cells per milliliter of milk is the indicator line ... less than 250,000 indicates a 'normal' condition, whereas above 250,000 indicates a degree of infection. In the United States the upper limit of the SCC allowed in milk sold to the public is 750,000 cells per milliliter of milk (except for Califormia, which has a 600,000 limit). One fluid ounce of milk equals 29.6 mililiters. This equates to 22.2 million cells per ounce of milk, or 177.6 million cells per 8 ounce serving. In Canada the upper limit is 500,000 cells per milliliter, in Europe it is 400,000.

The U.S. FDA supports the higher limit of 750,000 because, they argue, there is no known harmful effect to humans up to this level. Regulatory agencies in other countries disagree. It has been known for some time that the SCC of 750,000 is a strong indicator of an existing mastitis condition in the dairy cow. One much referenced study completed in 1995 concluded that an SCC of 750,000 indicates that 24.3% of the milked herd had a mastitis condition (Smith, 1995).

Regardless of the use of the somatic cell count as an indicator of mammary infection, many people are concerned about the presence of the somatic, or dead white blood cells themselves. If this is 'pus', then this itself is a matter of concern, they reason. The question then arises: "How much 'pus' is 750,000 cells per milliliter of milk ??" ... "How can it be measured, or visualized ??" To answer that question, and put it in perspective of, say, an 8 ounce glass of milk, let's do a little mathematical calculation. First, to get an idea of the physical size of a white blood cell, you could consider it to be roughly a sphere, about 10 μm in diameter. A 'μm' is one millionth of a meter, also called a 'micron'. If you were then to line up the somatic cells, bumper-to-bumper so to speak, 750,000 cells would extend 0.75 meters (or 75 centimeters, or 29.5 inches). The amount in an 8-ounce serving would then be 237 times that amount, or 177.8 meters (or about 583 feet).

However, this is unfair, because we are looking at only how long this would stretch out in a single linear line, but then this tiny thread of cells is only 10 μm in diameter, which is only 0.000393 inches, or approximately $1/2,600^{th}$ of an inch. So let's put this into a more tangible comparison. For example, consider the fabric threads that make up a good quality cloth, say with a thread count of 300 threads per inch. Then assume the individual thread to be round, the thread forming a long round bar. If the thread is $1/300^{th}$ of an inch in diameter, then it would be equivalent to 2,600 divided by 300 = 8.7 white blood cells, side to side. The cross sectional area would then occupy πr^2 number of cells, or 59 cells. Then, if you can picture this, each 8 ounce glass of milk, if the SCC is 750,000, would contain the amount of dead white corpuscles, or 'pus' equivalent in volume to a length of 583 divided by 59 = 9.9 feet of thread used in a 300 thread-count cloth. Finally, if you can imagine rolling that 9.9 feet length of that size of thread into a little ball, that is how much 'pus' you have in an 8 ounce glass of cow's milk with the maximum allowed SCC in the U.S.

Does commercial milk contain toxins?

A report by Tom Philpott of The Organic Center discloses test results conducted by the USDA in 2004 that showed some disturbing results:

"Ninety-six percent of samples contained DDE, "a breakdown product of DDT, which was banned from agricultural use in the early 1970s. DDT is very persistent and remains to this day in many cropland soils; its soil half-life (time required for 50 percent to dissipate) is generally between 15 and 30 years, depending on soil and climatic properties."

Nearly 99 percent contained diphenylamine (DPA), a "'high volume' industrial chemical used for many purposes in manufacturing rubber and plastic parts, and in making certain drugs."

Forty-one percent of samples contained dieldrin, a "long-banned" organochlorine pesticide. Endosulfan sulfate, an endocrine disrupter, turned up in 18 percent of samples.

About a quarter of samples delivered synthetic pyrethroid insecticides.

Nearly 9 percent of samples contained a chemical called 3-hydroxycarbofuran, a "highly-toxic breakdown product of the carbamate insecticide."

The USDA didn't comprehensively test conventional against organic milk. However, 10 of the 739 samples were labeled organic -- and "just like virtually all samples, all 10 samples contained DPA and nine had DDE residues," the Organic Center reports.

The good news is that the levels of DDE, DPA, and other pesticides found in milk in 2004 were very low. Most fell below one part per billion (ppb). The highest residue levels found were, at most, one-quarter of the applicable EPA tolerance (the maximum allowable limit of a pesticide in a given food)." (Philpott, 2008)

The USDA Pesticide Data Program concludes that pesticide residues in commercial milk do no reach risk levels. It may be significant to note that milk labeled 'organic milk' can contain the same levels of pesticide residues as non-organic milk, and sometimes even more. For example, Rusty Bishop of the Wisconsin Center for Dairy Research reports the following:

"The exposure of organic crops to synthetic pesticides is, indeed, less than that of conventional crops, but product results are somewhat variable and often mis-interpreted. USDA results from the Pesticide Data Program show no significant differences in pesticide levels between conventional and organic milk. Of the 739 milk samples tested, 100% contained low level pesticide residue, *all below actionable levels*. A similar survey in Italy concluded that organic and conventional samples of milk do not show relevant differences for organochlorine pesticides, PCBs, and heavy metals." (Bishop, 2007)

10. Does current food labeling tell us what is in our milk and milk products ... and how about false advertising?

Labeling

I remember a time when food labels simply stated the brand name and what it was ... that is, what it was mostly, or was supposed to be. And then it was required to list the main ingredients, and you could tell the relative amounts by the order in which they were listed. That was a revolutionary improvement. We have come a long ways since then ... but consumer awareness and concern has advanced even further, and faster. The dominant sentiment is now that we have a right to know what is in our foods ... accurately, precisely, and completely!

The dairy industry is one of the most regulated of all industries, and the laws governing the production, processing, and labeling of milk and milk products is one of the most advanced, compared with other foods. But there are still some important short-comings. The rBGH controversy has been discussed above, and labeling laws do not *require* that milk originating from treated cows be labeled as such. And Monsanto continues to lobby against legislation that would require such labeling, and *for* legislation that would prevent producers from labeling their milk or milk products as free from rBGH. The FDA still wrongly contends that there is no difference between milk from cows treated with rBGH and milk from untreated cows. This controversy is still ongoing and is an important matter of consumer concern.

As of 2006 the FDA requires that food labels clearly list any ingredients derived from any of the eight foods known to account for over 90% of documented food allergies in the U.S. Milk is the first on the list ... the remaining seven are eggs, fish, Crustacean shellfish, peanuts, tree nuts, wheat, and soybeans.

As noted in another section, labeling does not require notification of added lactose in any food product, thus placing the lactose intolerant individual at risk of developing digestive reactions without knowing that they have consumed lactose.

Milk and milk products may have high levels of contaminants, somatic cells, rBGH, anti-biotics, and even pesticides, all derived from the supplying animal ... but none of this is identified on milk labeling. The highly regulated production process protects against contaminants such as blood, manure, and feed particles, but a minute amount may still make it through the inspection and filtering. In the U.S. the maximum somatic cell count (SCC) is 750,000 per milliliter of milk, and this is regularly tested. The concern, however, is that the SCC is tested for at the time of pasteurization, and is therefore an average of all the milk from the many contributing cows making up the volume of milk in that one large storage tank ... some of the individual cows may have produced milk with a much higher SCC, which could potentially indicate a high state of disease in their udders. But this possiblility is hidden in the process. It is also of concern that the U.S. SCC standard is the highest of all major milk producing countries ... the maximum allowed SCC is 500,000 in Canada and 400,000 in Europe, Australia, and New Zealand. Several consumer advocacy groups have suggested that the U.S. lower the SCC maximum standard closer to that of the other countries.

The anti-biotic and pesticide level in milk is not required to be tested. Even if so, labeling requirements for pesticide content require that only 'active' ingredients need to be identified. So-called 'inert' chemicals are not required to be listed. However, these inert chemicals can also be harmful and may contribute to health problems. For example, some are known to be carcinogenic. It must be noted, however, that pesticides have not been found in any significant quantities in milk samples.

As of January 1, 2008, Pennsylvania law bans labels on milk and dairy products that say it comes from cows that haven't been treated with artificial bovine growth hormone (rBGH or rBST). The ban also extends to the use of phrases such as "pesticide free" and "antibiotic free". The reason stated is because (a) the labels are misleading and confusing to the consumer, (b) pesticide free and antibiotic free cannot be proven. (Now Public, 2010)

While with the FDA, Michael Taylor (noted above) was responsible for the creation of the "substantial equivalence" concept in reference to genetically modified crops and foods. Substantial equivalence assumes that a GM food is the same as its non-GM counterpart, and therefore requires no special testing, and, of course, no special labeling. However, research since then has shown that GM foods are indeed different from their non-GM equivalents. The Royal Society of Canada has described substantial equivalence as "scientifically unjustifiable and inconsistent with precautionary regulation of the technology". The UN FAO, WHO, and Codex Alimentarius also disagree with the concept and emphasize that safety assessment of GMOs must be focused on establishing the safety of new products. In 2001 the EU abandoned the doctrine of substantial equivalence in favor of more stringent scientific risk assessment. (Spin Profiles, 2010)

Current US labeling laws do not require that GM foods be identified as such on the labels.

False advertising

We have all seen the "Got Milk" and "milk mustache' ads ... and the heavy advertising that the dairy industry has engulfed us with as far back as we can remember. Even while in grade school many years ago I recall that much of our information about nutrition and what we should or should not eat was sponsored and made available through the dairy industry.

The Physicians Committee for Responsible Medicine has been an example of one effort to bring attention to misleading health claims in milk ads, and to campaign for government regulation. They explain their concerns in their newsletter:

"You've seen the ads: a celebrity dons a "milk mustache" and tells you to drink milk to ensure good health. With promises of strong bones, lower blood pressure, and better sports performance, these milk mustache ads are everywhere, providing millions of people with what unfortunately has become a primary source of nutritional information. But instead of helping, these ads are confusing and miseducating consumers. Most of the milk mustache ads that make health claims are false and misleading, and in violation of federal advertising guideline."

The PCRM continues to campaign for proper regulation. As far back as in the year 2000 the organization filed a petition with the Federal Trade Commission (FTC), requesting investigation of the milk mustache ads, which included those featuring Britney Spears, Marc Anthony, and Elton John; actors Jackie Chan and Noah Wyle; and athletes Serena and Venus Williams. It also explained why the U.S. Department of Agriculture's (USDA's) National Fluid Milk Processor Promotion Board, the dairy industry trade associations, and the advertising agency that developed the ad campaigns should all be held accountable for scientifically unsubstantiated, purposefully deceptive, and harmful advertising.

The petition was referred by the FTC to the USDA for investigation. But the irony ... and a case of political mischief ... is that it is the USDA that is promulgating these ads on behalf of the private dairy industry. (PCRM, 2010)

11. Calcium intake, lactose intolerance, and bone health ... a possible paradox ?

As I illustrated in the previous chapter, the greater majority of articles and research studies directed at osteoporosis emphasize the need for high calcium intakes to prevent or slow down bone loss, and dairy products are recommended as the best source of the required calcium. However, there seems to be a contradiction ... a paradox ... which is revealed in two startling statistics. One is that, worldwide, the populations that consume the highest amounts of calcium per capita, which also correlates with milk consumption, seem to be the same populations with the highest rates of osteoporosis. The Scandinavian countries drink the most milk and have the highest intakes of calcium, but they also have the highest rates of osteoporosis. The second statistic reveals that Native Americans, African-Americans, Asian-American, and Hispanic-American tend to be more lactose intolerant in this order, and therefore consume less dairy and obtain less calcium, yet have a lower incidence of osteoporosis ... apparently in the same order.

Are these conclusions justified ? What does science and objective analysis conclude about this apparent paradox ?

What is osteorporosis ?

Osteoporosis, literally meaning 'a porous condition' is a skeletal disease characterized by the deterioration of the architecture of bone tissue, and low bone density. The result is fragile bones and increased risk for fracture. Bone 'turnover', or absorption (formation) and resorption (breakdown) occurs throughout one's life, but it has been observed that it is normal for resorption to exceed absorption after reaching a peak density sometime between the ages of 30 to 40. Two types of osteoporosis are identified: type I is characterized by demineralization of mostly trabecular bone occurring mostly in post-menopausal women 50 to 65 years of age (about 10 to 15 years after menopause). Type II is characterized by demineralization of both cortical and trabecular bone, occurring in both men and women in later life, after 70 to 75 years.

The superb nutrition textbook, *Advanced Nutrition And Human Metabolism* (Gropper, Smith, and Groff, 2005) lists 11 factors critical to understanding and preventing osteoporosis, 8 of which are nutritional, and three of which relate to lifestyle or hormone function. I present these in the same order as listed in the text, with an explanation:

1. Estrogen. The female hormone, estrogen, has a positive effect on bone formation and mineralization, and is especially evidenced at puberty. A deficiency can cause bone resorption at any age, but is most prevalent after menopause. Estrogen replacement therapy (ERT) has been shown to improve bone density and reduce fracture risk with women after menopause. The treatment, however, is not without risk and is controversial.

2. Physical activity. The beneficial effect on bone mass by weight-bearing or weight-resistant exercise is well established. This may well be the most important single factor in preventing bone loss. Often cited examples of how effective exercise is include the example of tennis players, where it is commonly found that the bone density in their racket arm is significantly greater than in the other arm.

3. Calcium. Sufficient calcium during childhood, adolescence, and young adulthood has been found to be critical for attaining maximum peak bone density in the thirties.

4. Vitamin D. With the possible exception of digestion being assisted by lactose, vitamin D is essential in the absorption of calcium. Many studies have concluded that calcium *and* vitamin D must be provided together, and that vitamin D sometimes becomes the more critical nutrient.

5. Sodium. Sodium is excreted in the urine with calcium. For example, a sodium load of 100 mmol (2.3 grams) per day increases urinary calcium, measured from a baseline of no sodium intake, by 1 mmol (40 mg) per day. The question arises, however, as to where the calcium is coming from … is it only recently consumed calcium in the diet, or calcium from the blood, or calcium from the bone. Studies have arrived at different conclusions.

6. Phosphorus. Further research regarding the association of phosphorus and bone maintenance is urgently needed, but what is known is that high levels of phosphorus in the blood stimulates parathyroid hormone secretion, which then indirectly increases reabsorption of calcium by the renal tubules so that less calcium is lost in the urine. However, it is also known that phosphorus causes loss of calcium by increasing calcium secretion into the gastrointestinal tract, plus can stimulate increased blood concentrations at the expense of bone.

7. Protein. Adequate protein intake is necessary for bone health, and studies have shown that higher intakes of both protein and energy significantly improve recovery from bone fractures. However, protein in general, and especially the sulfur-containing amino acids methionine and

cystine (which may bind calcium) have been shown to increase calcium excretion.

8. Vitamins C and K. Both vitamins are important for the synthesis and function of various proteins found in bone, particularly collagen. Collagen is one of the main proteins found in bone, with vitamin C being the most critical vitamin requirement. Other proteins include osteocalcin and Gla protein, which cannot be synthesized without vitamin K. Low vitamin C and K intakes have been associated with an increased incidence of hip fractures in elderly men and women.

9. Fluoride. Although fluoride has been shown to reduce dental caries, high intakes fail to provide protection against osteoporosis, and may even be a causal factor.

10. Smoking. Smoking decreases circulating estrogen concentrations, thereby contributing to bone loss, and has been shown to be a significant predictor of bone loss in men.

11. Alcohol. The mechanisms by which alcohol exerts its effects are unclear but are thought to be multifactoral. Alcohol consumption has been significantly associated with increased rates of bone loss in men.

12. Caffeine. Caffeine reduces the renal reabsorption of calcium, which leads to increased urinary calcium losses. Although one cup of caffeinated coffee has been shown to promote an increase of only 6 mg of calcium in the urine, caffeine may also promote increased secretion of calcium into the gut. Caffeine intake has been positively associated with the risk of hip fractures in middle-aged women.

I would like to add that the following minerals are also known to be essential for bone metabolism: magnesium, zinc, manganese, iron, iodine, cobalt, molybdenum, vanadium, silicon, and boron. Additional vitamins involved include vitamins A, B-6, B-12, and D.

A critical lesson learned in nutrition is that none of the vitamins or minerals work alone ... it is important that *all* the essential nutrients are adequately supplied for any given body system to function properly. It is a mistake to concentrate on only one nutrient ... calcium for example, with the case of osteoporosis.

A review of the various publications on osteoporosis uncovers other factors related to the possible cause of this disease. One of note, from a National Osteoporosis Foundation fact sheet, suggests that thinness and smallness may be a contributing factor, which immediately makes me think of vegetarians. (NOF, 2010)

110

Another is genetics. A very recent study published in the Endocrine Review concludes that: "Genome-wide association studies have also identified common genetic variants of small size that contribute to regulation of BMD (bone mineral density) and fracture risk in the general population."

Yet another condition that is strongly associated with bone loss and the possible onset of osteoporosis is pregnancy and lactation. It is known that calcium delivered by the mother to the fetus or mammalian glands is sourced directly from the mother's blood, which then must be quickly replaced, directed by homeostatic functions. If the calcium isn't available from an immediate dietary intake, then it will be resorbed from bone. Lactation and pregnancy can therefore place direct and immediate stress on BMD (bone mineral density). (Ziegler, 1996)

Do the countries with the highest intake of calcium and dairy have the highest rates of osteoporosis?

There are a number of statistical analyses and studies that confirm that the countries with the highest intakes of calcium, which is usually highlighted by a corresponding high dairy intake, have the highest rates of osteoporosis. Is this true ? And is this therefore an argument that promoting high dairy and high calcium intakes is leading in the wrong direction?

Several studies and observations show that the answer is not a simple yes or no ... there are possible confounders and alternative explanations. I discuss these in the next sections.

Lack of statistics

Yes, available statistics point to a high intake of calcium, mostly obtained through consumption of milk, in Northern Europe, United States, and the UK. And yes, statistics show very high rates of osteoporosis as well. So the claim that the countries with the highest calcium and milk consumption are also the countries with the highest rates of osteoporosis, at first glance, seems plausible. And this would seem to expose an interesting paradox. However, one problem with this conclusion is that it is based on incomplete statistics ... only on statistics that were available several years ago. The reality is that we lack statistics for other countries, even now, and that the high rates of osteoporosis, particularly in the United States, are based on studies of mostly Caucasian subjects. The most recent statistics do *not* support the conclusion that the countries with the highest rates of osteoporosis also have the highest intakes of dairy and calcium.

Using Asia as an example, the International Osteoporosis Foundation's 2010 updated statistics and statements include the following:

"It is projected that more than about 50% of all osteoporotic hip fractures (in the world) will occur in Asia by the year 2050."

"Osteoporosis is greatly underdiagnosed and undertreated in Asia, even in the most high risk patients who have already fractured. The problem is particularly acute in rural areas. In the most populace countries like China and India, the majority of the population lives in rural areas (80% in China) where hip fractures are often treated conservatively at home instead of by surgical treatment in hospitals."

"DXA technology is relatively expensive and not widely available in Asian countries."

"Nearly all Asian countries fall far below the FAO/WHO recommendations for calcium intake of between 1000 and 1300 mg/day. The median dietary calcium intake for the adult Asian population is approximately 450 mg/day."

"Studies carried out across different countries in South and South East Asia showed, with few exceptions, widespread prevalence of vitamin D deficiency/insufficiency, in both sexes and in all age groups of the population." (IOF, 2010)

The *China Study* by Colin Campbell is used as one reference to support the paradox theory, in which he states that the incidence of bone fractures in China is one-fifth that of in the U.S. However, it seems that this conclusion is based on incomplete and outdated statistics. For China, the IOF 2010 update states the following:

"Osteoporosis affects almost 70 million Chinese over the age of 50 and causes some 687,000 hip fractures in China each year."

"Osteoporosis prevention and awareness is largely restricted to urban areas of China and DXA machines are only available in the urban centers."

"Hong Kong, China: Epidemiological studies showed that hip fracture incidence had increased by 300% from the 1960s to 1990s, and has stabilized from 2001 – 2008. The reasons are not clear, but may possibly be due to a number of factors including improved availability of medical intervention, increases in BMI (body weight), use of HRT (heat treatment in milk production), and improved falls prevention strategies."

"Hong Kong, China: The prevalence of vertebral fractures is estimated at 30% in women and 17% in men between the ages of 70 – 79. These rates are comparable to those in American Caucasians." (IOF, 2010)

An excellent example of the osteoporosis situation in Asian countries, and perhaps for Africa and South America as well, is the case of Thailand. When I was studying at the University of Mahidol at the Salaya campus, on the north-west outskirts of Bangkok, I became intimately involved in the study of Thailand's nutritional problems. The story of Thailand's emergence from an 'underdeveloped' to a 'developing country', with a heavy health burden, is a remarkable success story. For example, as recent as 1981 the country experienced a measured population-wide malnutrion rate of 52%, but was able to reduce that to 21% within 5 years.

Prior to the late 1990s osteoporosis was not on the priority list of disease conditions to be addressed by the Thai Department of Health and the professional nutritionists working at the Department of Health or teaching/researching at the several top-ranking universities, such as Mahidol and Chulalongkorn, and statistics did not begin to emerge until after the year 2000. We did know that typical calcium intakes were low … about 600 mg per day, and we knew that osteoporosis conditions were common, although not paid much attention to nor measured. There were no national or regional figures giving the prevalence of osteoporosis and no standard normal curve for Thai bone mineral densities (BMD). In the year 2000 only six of the nation's 76 provinces possessed even a single 'bone densitometer'. Although there were no statistics on the prevalence of osteoporosis, I could observe a good number of older men, and especially older women, with bent-over bodies and sharply deformed upper- spine curvatures.

While at Mahidol the promotion of milk and dairy products was a hot topic. Prior to the 90s almost no milk or its derivatives was consumed in Thailand. But the nutritionists that were my *ajaan* (professors) and who worked in the Thai Department of Health were all trained in universities in the U.S., Australia, or Europe. My advisor, for example, gained her PhD from Cornell, and the newly appointed director of the Institute of Nutrion at Mahidol University (INMU) at the time, Ajaan Emorn, earned her PhD from the Massachusetts Institute of Technology, and her mentor there had been no other than the internationally renowned Dr. Nevin Scrimshaw. These western-trained nutritionists, deeply ingrained in the

113

conventional wisdom of the countries where they received their degrees, of course wanted to promote the consumption of milk and dairy products. As mentioned, the average adult intake of calcium in the 90s was estimated to be about 600 mg/day. And almost all Thai had become indoctrinated to believing that 'milk' was the key to growing tall and having strong bones. A delightful young Thai lady once told me that "she was very angry at her mother … because she had not given her milk as a youngster, and that was why she was so short". It was a common belief. And a good percentage of Thais did, indeed, try to consume milk. It was common that they could drink perhaps 6 to 8 ounces a day with no or little lactase insufficiency problems. Yogurt also became popular. Cheese ?? … no … very few Thais will eat cheese, even in the year 2010. So milk and milk products are consumed, but only minimally.

Even with a greater availability of meat and meat products, the Thai remain basically vegetarian. Chicken and pork are commonly consumed daily in small quantities, but almost no beef. A typical modern plate is stilled based on rice.

The very first Thai study on the prevalence of osteoporosis was carried out in 2001 by Limpaphayom et al. I am sad to report that the study scientists came from Chulalongkorn University, not my Institute of Nutrition at Mahidol. The study subjects consisted of 1,935 Thai women aged 40 – 80 years, with random selection and multistage sampling and stratifying from 6 provinces. Their conclusion: "Using the Thai BMD reference, the age-specific prevalence of osteoporosis among Thai women rose progressively with increasing age to more than 50% after the age of 70." (Limpaphayom et al, 2001)   This is a surprisingly high rate, even exceeding that established by most studies for American Caucasians.

The argument that world-wide global rates show a strong correlation of high calcium intakes with high rates of osteoporosis is not therefore supported by more recent statistics and recent studies.

Possible 'confounders' … vitamin D, latitiude, and skin-coloring

The cases of countries occupying areas in the higher latitudes of Europe may be unique, and the research results may be influenced by strong 'confounders'. A 'confounder' is a factor that can be a possible separate cause from the one being identified, the inter-play of which may render the original analysis totally invalid. As I have discussed in Chapter One and Two, Northern Europeans faced special challenges when trying to fulfill their need for calcium, and acquired special adaptations. This centered on the need for vitamin D, essential for absorbing and utilizing calcium. Two related factors are critical for people living in high latitudes: the first is the lack of sunlight to synthesized vitamin D in the skin, and the second is the presence or relative non-presence of ultra-violet-blocking melanin in the skin. As explained in Chapter Two, it is known that low levels of sunlight will inhibit the amount of the provitamin D synthesized. For example, the amount of sunshine available during the months of November through February at a latitude equivalent to the city of Boston is insufficient to produce significant vitamin D synthesis (Human Nutrition, pp 415). The latitude of Boston is 41.78 degrees ... London is 51.32, Dublin 53.20, Stockholm 59.17, and Oslo 59.55. Studies have shown a strikingly close correlation of latitude with the incidence of osteoporosis, and conclude that latitude and the resulting inability to synthesize provitamin D has a strong association with the risk for osteoporosis, and may be a confounder for the high rate of calcium/high rate of osteoporosis hypothesis.

A common observation related to this discussion is that the UK and the Scandinavian countries now have a substantial and increasing presence of darker-skinned persons due to heavy in-migration from African, Asian, and Middle-East countries. It is known that these people are particularly susceptible to vitamin D insufficiency due to the lack of sunlight at higher latitudes, and may account for an increased incidence of osteoporosis nation-wide ... although I know of no study that addresses this possibility.

In the case of the Eskimo and the seeming paradox of a high intake of calcium combined with a high rate of osteoporosis, a possible confounder may be the known relationship of vitamin D toxicity with bone loss. Eskimos consume a very large amount of fish oils rich in pre-formed vitamin D. I know of no research on this topic, but excess vitamin D obtained from a high intake of fish oils could be a possible confounder to the hypothesis that a high intake of calcium from fish bone is correlated with a high risk of osteoporosis. The possibility that the calcium from fish bone is not bioavailable could also be a confounder.

Do all ethnic and nationality groups have the same requirement for calcium?

A recent report by the United Nation's World Health Organization (WHO) makes the following statement:

"The report of the Joint FAO/WHO Expert Consultation on Vitamin and Mineral Requirements in Human Nutrition made it clear that the recommendations for calcium intakes were based on long-term (90 days) calcium balance data for adults derived from Australia, Canada, the European Union, the United Kingdom, and the United States, and were not necessarily applicable to all countries worldwide. The report also acknowledged that strong evidence was emerging that the requirement for calcium might vary from culture to culture for dietary, genetic, lifestyle and geographical reasons." (WHO, 2010)

. John Robbins references a study of African Bantu women who take in only 350 mg of calcium per day, yet bear an average of nine children, breast feed them for two full years, and yet seldom break a bone and rarely lose a tooth.

There is, therefore, evidence that non-white ethnic groups have lower rates of osteoporosis and do not require the same levels of calcium intake. This suggests that the associated need for calcium in the prevention of osteoporosis is not universal, or consistant. This observation could then help explain why Northern Europeans tend to have higher rates of osteoporosis, even with higher intakes of calcium.

The assertion that there is a paradox between high dairy and calcium intake with osteoporosis can therefore be seen as a complex issue that remains controversial. The observation that countries that have the highest intakes of dairy and calcium are also the countries with the highest rates of osteoporosis may be confounded by (a) a lack of statistics for other countries, (b) availability of vitamin D, associated with latitiude, and (c) the possibility that Northern Europeans are ethnically more susceptible for osteoporosis. Bioavailability of calcium from specific sources may be another factor. The finding that non-white ethnic groups may have less need for calcium, demonstrated by a lower incidence of osteoporosis along with lower dairy and calcium intakes, is less controversial, however. But this does not mean that a paradox exists, only that the assumption that all peoples have the same requirement for calcium may be invalid.

Osteoporosis and the vegetarian point of view

In the last few years proponents of the new anti-milk movement have picked-up on the apparent contradiction between high dairy and calcium intakes coupled with high rates of osteoporosis, and have become very vocal … especially writers from the pro-vegetarian camp. Two central arguments have been proposed, which are (1) that the recommended daily intakes of calcium are much higher than needed and is a result of advertising and marketing by the dairy industry, and (2) that the real culprit is not inadequate intakes of calcium, but is instead due to consuming too much *protein*, which causes calcium to (a) be excreted in the urine, or (b) causes an acidic condition in the body and calcium is then resorbed from bone mass to use as an alkaline buffer.

John Robbins, author of two very popular books, *Diet For A New America (1987)* and *The Food Revolution: How Your Diet Can Help Save Your Life And The World* is a strong advocate of vegetarianism and references evidence that calcium intake does not correlate with the rate of osteoporosis among world populations. He cites the fairly well-known observation that the United States, Finland, Sweden, and the United Kingdom consume the largest quantity of dairy products (and the highest intakes of calcium) and yet have the highest rates of osteoporosis. Further, he notes that native Eskimos consume more than 2000 mg of calcium a day in the form of fish bones, yet have one of the very highest rates of osteoporosis. Jane Plant, for instance, writes: "Countries with the highest consumption of dairy products have the highest bone fracture rates. In countries like China and Nigeria, where they have very little dairy and much less calcium, their rates of osteoporosis are about 200 times less than the UK's." (Plant, 2003)

Recommended intakes for calcium may be too high ?

One prominent ant-milk website, www.milksucks.com, quotes Dr. T. Colin Campbell, author of *The China Study: The Most Comprhensive Study of Nutrition Ever Conducted and the Startling Implications for Diet, Weight Loss and Long Term Health* (2004) and founder of the "T. Colin Campbell Foundation, Scientific Integrity for Optimal Health":

"The dairy folks, ever since the 1920s, have been enormously successful in cultivating an environment within virtually all segments of our society – from research and education to public relations and politics – to have us believing that cow's milk and its products are manna from heaven. … Make no mistake about it; the dairy industry has been virtually in total control of any and all public health information that ever rises to the level of public scrutiny.

Jane Plant, in her recent book *Understanding, Preventing, and Overcoming Osteoporosis* (2003), concludes:

"It goes against conventional belief, but medical experts now believe that extra calcium from dairy is only important while your bodies are forming during childhood and adolescence. Obviously, you still need some calcium for your body and bones to stay healthy and it may be worth including more healthy dairy-free sources in your diet, such as hazelnuts, egg yolks, brazil nuts, green olives, figs – even oranges."

Not inadequate intakes of calcium, but instead too much *protein* ... calcium loss and acid-base imbalance ?

Robbins and others in the same camp, notably John A. McDougall, author of 12 books on nutrition, theorize that osteoporosis is not caused by a deficiency of calcium, but rather by an excessive loss of calcium due to a high intake of animal protein. Dr. McDougall is quoted as stating:

"I would like to emphasize that the calcium-losing effect of protein on the human body is not an area of controversy in scientific circles. The many studies performed during the past 55 years consistently show that the most important dietary change that we can make if we want to create a positive calcium balance that will keep our bones solid is to decrease the amount of proteins we eat each day. The important change is not to increase the amount of calcium we take in." (Robbins, *The Truth About Calcium and Osteoporosis*)

Therefor, upon reviewing the theoretical basis for which bone calcium is lost, according to Robbins, McDougall, Keon, Plant, and others of the same viewpoint, two mechanisms are identified. One is the observed promotion of calcium loss in the urine with increased protein intake, particularly the sulfur-containing amino acids. The second is a theoretical homeostatic resorption (breakdown) of alkaline calcium from the bone to neutralize excessive acidity in the blood caused by, again, a high intake of protein ... this is the "acid-base imbalance caused by high protein hypothesis".

The first mechanism is verified from many studies and nutrition textbooks. It is known that intakes of protein can correspond with urinary losses of calcium in a ratio as high as 1.7 mg of calcium for every gram of protein ingested. This means that a protein intake increase of 20 grams can result in a calcium urinary loss of as much as 34 mg.

The second mechanism involves the much-discussed acid-base imbalance hypothesis. The vegetarian author, Joseph Keon, in his book *Whole Health* (1997), summarizes the argument as follows:

"The truth is, it is important to look at how much calcium one retains, rather than what one consumes. When we compare worldwide rate of osteoporosis, we see that the disease is relatively rare in places where protein is consumed in moderate amounts. Conversely, countries with the highest rates of osteoporosis (Norway, Sweden, and Denmark) also have the highest intakes of animal proteins. Why is this? High levels of protein result in more acidic blood. In an effort to buffer this acid and achieve a more appropriate blood balance, the body utilizes calcium, eventually drawing on the calcium stored in the bones, a process known as 'calcium leaching'."

The counter-vegetarian point of view

The previous three sections have presented the point of view regarding osteoporosis widely promoted by the vegetarian community. Their reasoning and supportive evidence, however, is highly suspect. I have observed the development of the vegetarian logic for many years, and conclude that the primary motive for their peculiar conclusions is to support the premise that we do not need as much protein as recommended. Why? Simply because it is very difficult to obtain recommended levels of protein intake on a vegetarian diet, especially a vegan diet … and especially 'complete' protein.

In the next five sections I will present the science and reasoning that counters the vegetarian view.

Historical perspective of calcium intakes

Calcium intake by humans can be viewed from a historical perspective. Prior to the 20th century and going back for several hundred years, perhaps even a few thousand, it is clear that our forefathers consumed a lot less calcium than more contemporary man. I remember that Alan Lad was popularly selected for movie roles as a medieval knight because his small stature allowed him to fit into the armor preserved from that era. Anthropometric history tells us that the average height of 4th century Europeans was about 5 ft. 5 in. (165 centimeters). The average height of the confederate soldier in the great American Civil War was 5 ft 6 in. Height is influenced by a number of factors, but nutrition is important, and calcium intake is one of the more critical nutrients. S. Boyd Eaton, the pioneer and noted expert on the diet and nutritional status of early man tells us that the Paleolithic diet provided double the calcium intake of modern man, and that with the advent of agriculture and the domestication of animals and food plants man's average height dropped 6 inches. He remarks that only now is man's height re-approaching that of pre-agricultural hunters and gatherers.

"The nutritional requirements of contemporary humans were almost certainly established over eons of evolutionary experience and the best available evidence indicates that this evolution occurred in a high-calcium nutritional environment. The exercise and dietary patterns of humans living at the end of the Stone Age can be considered natural paradigms: calcium intake was twice that for contemporary humans and requirements for physical exertion were also greater than at present. Bony remains from that period suggest that Stone Agers developed a greater peak bone mass and experienced less age-related bone loss than do humans in the 20th Century." (Eaton and Nelson, 1991)

If taken seriously, this suggests that our currently recommended calcium intakes fall far short of what our physiologies were designed for. It also suggests that disease conditions such as osteoporosis must be viewed in this light, as well.

Other considerations in this context include the availability and intake of other nutrients ... even protein, for example. Our forefathers of that era consumed as much as three times the protein that we do now.

High protein causes urinary loss of calcium

First and foremost, in all the readings and research that I have done on the subject of osteoporosis, there have been no credible studies which conclude that high protein intake is directly associated with osteoporosis, although some studies *do* identify an association with low protein intakes.

However, it *is* known that dietary protein intakes can influence calcium urinary loss, but this has not been shown to significantly influence long-term calcium resorption from bone. One of my most highly regarded university textbooks sums this issue up as follows:

"Although studies over the past half century established that high amounts of dietary protein taken as an isolated nutrient increase renal calcium excretion, epidemiological studies showed no adverse effect of high amounts of dietary protein on either the rate of hip fractures or metacarpal cortical bone mass." (Arnaud and Sanchez, 1996)

Never-the-less, just for the sake of argument, let's take the argument presented by proponents such as John McDougall, John Robbins, and Colin Campbell seriously for a moment. Tests have shown that intakes of protein can influence calcium excretion in the urine up to 1.7 mg. for each gram of protein ingested. This means that if one was to increase their protein intake from, say, 30 grams per day (an amount consumed by many vegetarians) to 51 grams per day (the RDA average for all American adults), this could possibly increase calcium excretion in the urine as much as 1.7 x 21 = 36 mg, all other things equal. Now, if the recommended intake of the same average adult is 1,000 mg, and the absorption rate is 30%, then this would lower the 333 mg of available calcium by 10.8%, to 297 mg. of calcium. Is this a significant loss? I suggest that it is not. Then, we must also ask where the calcium that is excreted comes from … is it calcium that is digested at the same meal as the protein, or is it calcium in the blood stream, or is it truly calcium that has been resorbed from the body's bone mass, or as has been suggested, is *leached* from the bone, due only to the digestion of protein in a given meal?

In order to shed some science to the discussion, I would like to quote two paragraphs from another favorite text book:

"Calcium is excreted in the urine and feces, although up to182 mg (average, 60 mg) may be lost daily from the skin, especially with extreme sweating. Most calcium is filtered and reabsorbed by the kidneys such that urinary calcium losses range from about 100 to 240 mg per day, with an average of about 170 mg. Urinary calcium excretion may be decreased by PTH secretion as well as in the presence of phosphorus, potassium, magnesium, and boron, and it may be increased in the presence of sodium, protein, boron plus magnesium, and caffeine.

Fecal losses of calcium from endogenous sources range from about 45 to 100 mg per day. Fecal loses may increase with consumption of fiber, phytate, and oxalate, and of magnesium in excess, and in people with fat-malabsorbing disorders." (Gropper, Smith, and Groff, 2005, pp 389)

This illustrates that calcium is actively absorbed, is lost via the skin, in the urine, and in feces, and is also reabsorbed (re-cycled) by the kidneys. This is all a normal process, and occurs every day. Of the approximate 330 mg that is successfully absorbed from an RDA amount of 1,000 mg, 18 – 55% can be lost through the skin via sweating, 30 – 73% through the urine, and 14 – 30% lost in fecal matter. What is important in all of this is the *net* gain or loss. The urinary loss of calcium due to protein intake is not likely to be significant in relation to osteoporosis, as is shown by the findings that high protein intake is *not* associated with bone loss or fractures.

Perhaps the most credible study in this respect is the landmark study of diet and bone in the Framingham Osteoporosis Study, which was conducted as part of the famous Framingham Heart Study. The conclusions of Tucker et al included:

> "In contrast to the hypothesis (that high protein intak causes bone loss), we did not find that higher protein intakes lead to greater bone loss. Rather, we found that those with the greatest protein intakes in this study had the highest BMD ... contrary to expectations, we found that elders with the highest intake of total protein and of animal protein had the least bone loss after controlling for known confounders. Rather than causing bone loss, as was hypothesized, animal protein intake appeared to be important in maintaining bone of minimizing bone loss in elderly persons." (Tucker et al, *The acid-base hypothesis: diet and bone in the Framingham Osteoporosis Study,* 2001)

In summary, the notion that higher intakes of protein contribute to osteoporosis is not supported by recent scientific investigation, and the notion truly borders on the absurd.

Protein and calcium loss ... the acid-base imbalance hypothesis

The second claim from the vegetarian camp regarding protein, as noted, is that proteins are acidic and the body therefore must work to offset the increased acidity caused by intakes of high amounts of proteins, and calcium resorbed from the bone is used for this purpose, thus causing a loss of calcium from the bone.

A survey of recent studies indicate that this is a highly controversial conclusion. There is evidence that consuming foods that result in a more acidic environment within the body *can* as a consequence promote resorption of calcium from bone and lead to loss of bone mass. It is important to understand that the propensity of a given food to contribute to increased acidity or alkalinity in the body is not necessarily its measure of its acidity or alkalinity in its state prior to ingestion. As John Berardi explains,

"When a food is ingested, digested, and absorbed, each component of that food will present itself to the kidneys as either an acid-forming compound or a base-forming one (alkaline). And when the sum total of all the acid producing and the base producing micro and macronutrients is tabulated (at the end of a meal or at the end of a day), we're left with a calculated acid-base load. If the diet provides more acidic components, it will obviously manifest as a net-acid load on the body. And if it provides more basic components, it will obviously manifest as a net base load on the body."

The acid-base hypothesis has been around for a long time, and has been much discussed from various perspectives for at least 100 years. Paleolithic diet enthusiasts have recently pointed out that our modern diet, especially in the post-industrial revolution era, has leaned towards increased acid producing foods, largely as a result of consuming dairy and grain products. One of the leaders in this debate is T. Remer, who published *Potential renal acid load of foods and its influence on urine pH.* (Remer, 1995), in which he calculated a "potential renal acid load per 100 grams" scale (PRAL) for 114 different foods. In his scale, a positive number indicates acidity, and a negative number indicates alkalinity (base), the higher the number the more acidic or alkaline.

Milk and dairy products are markedly acidic, especially cheeses. The most acidic food on the entire list is Parmesan cheese, with a score of +34.2, followed closely by other cheeses. Other milk products are much less acid producing, ranging on the scale from 0.7 for pasteurized whole milk to 1.5 for whole milk yogurt.

Grains and grain products range from 1.7 for boiled white rice to 8.2 for whole wheat flour and 12.6 for brown rice. Whole eggs are 8.2, egg yolk is 23.4.

Meat and meat products go from 6.7 for frankfurters to 7.8 for lean beef, 7.9 for pork, 8.7 for chicken, and 13.2 for canned corned beef (high mostly due to salt content).

Fish is acidic, ranging from 6.8 for haddock to 10.8 for trout. Nuts *can* be acidic (walnuts 6.8) or alkaline (hazelnuts –2.8). Legumes can also be both acidic (peanuts 8.3) and alkaline (green beans -3.1). Fats and oils tend to be neutral, with sugar and honey slightly alkaline.

All common beverages tend to be alkaline or near neutral, with beer averaging 0.2, wines -1.8, coffee -1.4, coca-cola 0.4, and cocoa -0.4.

All fruits are alkaline, ranging from an extreme of -21.0 for raisins, -2.9 for orange juice, to -1.0 for grape juice.

All vegetables are also alkaline, as alkaline as -14.0 for spinach to -4.9 for carrots, and -0.4 for asparagus. (Remer, 1995)

Pertinent to this discussion is the conclusion by some observers and researchers that a net acid load at the kidneys will result in resorption of calcium from bone to the kidneys to neutralize the acidity.

This is a curious proposition.

Now, it is true that the acid-base balance in the body must be tightly controlled within a narrow range. As stated in the textbook *Advanced Nutrition and Human Metabolism (Gropper, Smith, and Groff, 2005):*

> " its regulation is one of the most important aspects of homeostasis, because merely slight deviations from normal acidity can cause marked alteration in enzyme-catalyzed reaction rates in the cells. ... The degree of acidity of any fluid is determined by its concentration of protons (H^+)."

To guard against fluctuations in pH, three principal regulatory systems are available:

> "Buffer systems within the fluids that immediately neutralize acidic or basic compounds; the respiratory center, which regulates breathing and the rate of exhalation of CO_2; and renal regulation, by which acidic or alkaline urine can be formed to adjust body fluid acidity."

The respiratory system, of course, has nothing to do with either protein intake or calcium resorption. The buffer system also has nothing to do with calcium resorption. In fact, the chief buffers used by the body for acid-base balance are proteins.

> "Proteins, because of their constituent amino acids, can serve as a buffer in the body. A buffer is a compound that ameliorates a change in pH that would otherwise occur in response to the addition of alkali or acid to a solution. The pH of the blood and other body tissues must be maintained within an appropriate range. Blood pH ranges from about 7.35 to 7.45, whereas cellular pH of red blood cells is about 7.2, and that of muscle cells is about 6.9. The H^+ concentration within cells is buffered by both the phosphate system and the amino acids in proteins. The protein hemoglobin, for example, functions as a buffer in red blood cells. In the plasma and extracellular fluid, proteins and the bicarbonate system serve as buffers. Amino acids act as acids or bases in aqueous solutions such as those in the body by releasing and accepting hydrogen ions, thereby contributing to the buffering capacity of proteins in the body."

Now, how about renal regulation of pH (regulation of acid or alkali changes by the kidneys)? Perhaps this is where calcium might have a role. But we find that this is not so:

"The kidneys regulate pH by controlling the secretion of hydrogen ions, by conserving or producing bicarbonate, and by synthesizing the ammonia from glutamine (an amino acid) to form ammonium ions. The secretion of hydrogen ions occurs in conjunction with the tubular reabsorption of sodium ions."

Calcium does not, therefore, normally play a role in maintaining the body's acid-base balance homeostasis.

Vegetarian foods can also be acidic ...

For the sake of argument, is should be noted that many foods accepted in the vegetarian diet are highly acidic. Yes, it is true that all fruits and vegetables are alkaline, with negative PRAL values. However, if the individual includes dairy products in their vegetarian diet, then they will consume cheese, which has the highest of all PRAL values. If they include fish and eggs, they will also be consuming moderately high PRAL foods ... the average PRAL for fish is 7.9 and 8.2 for whole eggs. Even if they are strict vegans, a number of accepted vegan foods have high PRAL ratings. Brown rice has a PRAL of 12.5, rolled oats 10.7, peanuts 8.3, whole wheat flour 8.2, whole grain spaghetti 7.3, and cornflakes 6.0. These are all comparable to the PRALs of red meats (average 8.2) and poultry (average 9.3). The claim that proteins from animal foods have a higher PRAL is therefore only partially justified. Plus, there is no distinction one way or another whether the protein source is animal or vegetable. This makes sense ... proteins are comprised of amino acids, and, for example, a lysine amino acid is a lysine amino acid ... there is no difference in its structure whether it comes as part of a vegetable or as part of red meat ... and during digestion the protein is separated into its component amino acids, and it is the individual amino acids that transport across the intestinal membrane ... whole proteins are too large to transport across.

What ... then ... makes a food acidic or alkaline ?

A useful analogy is to think of the metabolic utilization of a given food substance as a *burning* process, leaving an *ash*, or mineral residue. Alkaline ash consists of the minerals sodium, potassium, calcium, and magnesium. Acidic ash is mostly composed of sulfur, phosphorus, chlorine, and organic acidic radicals. Acidity and alkalinity are measured with the pH scale, 0 being the maximum acidic, 14 the maximum alkaline, and 7.0 being neutral. A food may have been very acidic, with a low pH before ingestion, but becomes alkaline when metabolized. An example is the lemon, which is very acidic with a pH in the neighborhood of 3 ... similar to the acidity of stomach juices ... but when metabolized becomes one of the most alkaline of all the fruits.

Research has shown that supplementation of the appropriate minerals can contribute significantly to net acidity or alkalinity. For example, supplemental intake of calcium, potassium, and/or magnesium can promote alkalinity, or offset the acid effect of acid-producing foods.

However, an effect on the net acid excretion (NAE) at the kidneys does not necessarily translate to calcium resorption from the bone and a lower bone mineral density (BMD). One very recent meta-analysis of 16 previous studies is particularly revealing. The 16 studies were collected by a systematic search of published literature ... each had concluded that an association existed between the consumption of protein and grain foods with increased urine calcium and release of calcium from the skeleton. Only five of the studies were randomized and met the quality criteria of the Institute of Medicine's Panel on Calcium and Related Nutrients for calcium studies. The meta-analysis of the five surviving studies showed no relationship between a change of net acid excretion (NAE) and a change in calcium balance. There was also no relationship between a change of NAE and a change in the marker of bone metabolism.

> "In conclusion, this meta-analysis does not support the concept that the calciuria associated with higher NAE reflects a net loss of whole body calcium. There is no evidence from superior quality balance studies that increasing the diet acid load promotes skeletal bone mineral loss or osteoporosis. Changes of urine calcium do not accurately represent calcium balance. Promotion of the "alkaline diet" to prevent calcium loss is not justified." (Fenton et al, 2009)

In fairness, it must also be reported that the study referenced above by Tucker et al (*The acid-base hypothesis: diet and bone in the Framingham Osteoporosis Study*), although *not* supporting the hypothesis that high protein intake promotes bone loss, they did find weak evidence that the intake of alkaline foods and minerals is associated with less bone loss in the elderly. In the results section entitled *Effect of baseline magnesium, potassium and fruit and vegetable intake on subsequent four-year change in BMD*, they conclude

"Among men, greater baseline potassium intake was significantly associated with lower subsequent four-year loss in BMD at the femoral neck and trochanter. Magnesium intake was significantly associated with subsequent change in BMD at the femoral neck and trochanter, and approached significance at Ward's area. The combined potassium + magnesium z-score was significant for the femoral neck and trochanter, and Ward's area. Fruit and vegetable intake approached significance at the trochanter and was significant at Ward's area ... none of the longitudinal results for women were significant." (Tucker et al, 2001)

Non-dairy sources of calcium

There is no question that cow's milk is an excellent source of calcium, and it is difficult to meet the RDA requirements from plant foods, as I've shown in the table entitled Calcium Content of Selected Plant Foods in the section on vegetarianism. It is also generally true that meats and fish are not good sources of calcium. However, there *are* good sources of calcium if we select the most calcium-dense plant foods and add a few other alternatives. Soybeans are particulary calcium-dense, and tofu, made from soybeans, is an even better source because it is usually prepared with calcium sulfate and magnesium (nigari). Because we normally eat the bones of the small sardine, this is also a food high in calcium. Tortilla corn flour is normally treated with lime, containing calcium carbonate, and so tortillas also have a high calcium content. A small number of commonly consumed fish have substantial calcium as well, rainbow trout and halibut, for example. In addition, calcium is being added as a fortification in an increasing number of foods. Orange juice, for example. The form of calcium added in orange juice is calcium citrate. Most of the research studies on bioavailability of the various forms of calcium do not conclude that calcium citrate, calcium sulfate, or forms other than calcium carbonate, which is the form in cow's milk, is digested any easier or is utilized any more efficiently. However, I suspect some mischief in this respect. Calcium carbonate is easily the most common form of calcium on the planet, being the substance of coral, the sand at the ocean-side beach, the stuff utilized in plaster, gypsum, and concrete, and in mountains of limestone. All this also suggests that maybe calcium carbonate is not so suitable for roles in human biology.

There are a few studies which show that other forms, particularly calcium citrate, are more bioavailable (Reinwald, 2008). One other study introduced the novel concept that supplementation with calcium-rich mineral water was an effective way of supplementing calcium (Bohmer, 2000).

There is also the option of using supplements. Here I have another story to tell. Because I cannot handle milk very well due to lactose intolerance, I have always been aware that I need to actively seek sources other than milk for my calcium, and almost for the entire duration of my adult life I have taken calcium supplements. My older sister's son, Vince, has had an even more serious problem in this respect. For most of his younger years he was intolerant to milk to the point of being outright allergic. A single glass of milk would cause him to break out in hives.

Now Vince is an interesting subject !! Vince was born club-footed. Kinda severely so. And Vince loves motorcycles, and was active in motor-cross racing way back when it was a brand-new sport. During one event Vince broke his ankle, and, low and behold, when the doctor braced his leg and ankle, he was able to correct that club-foot condition … at least on that side. Then, later, Vince was involved in another mishap and broke the other ankle. Again the doctor was able to place the braces so to correct the club-foot problem on that side as well. Maybe having low bone density due to not being able to drink milk had something to do with it. Maybe not. But then, when Vince was in his early forties he smashed up his brand-new Harley and really messed himself up, with multiple leg and hip fractures. It was then discovered that he did, indeed, have low bone density, and this was now a severe disability. Well, Vince had been around my mother's health food store, located in Osoyoos, in southern British Columbia when Vince was growing up in Kerameos, a few miles away. So he knew about supplements. He experimented with various brands and combinations, and then discovered 'Bone-Up' made by Jarrow, then an exclusively Australian company. His doctor was surprised to notice that Vince's bone density was suddenly increasing. "This is not supposed to be happening !!" he told Vince. "What have you been taking ??" Vince told him. And now Doctor Y recommends Bone Up to all his patients. Hush-hush, of course … for he is bound by protocol, his hospital and peers, and his pharmaceutical supplier.

This brings me to a key issue, and question. Our conventional wisdom stresses calcium as the key nutrient for supporting and maintaining our bone mass. And in the little that mainstream medicine ventures into the world of supplements, a calcium supplement is just that … a calcium supplement. But we know that bone growth and maintenance requires a number of nutrients in addition to calcium, and so the question arises: "Why are supplements recommended to enhance bone growth and maintenance contain only calcium?" The folks who are bold enough to explore this question come up with a very different view and recommendation. In addition to 1000 mg of calcium, Bone Up, for example, contains 200 mg of vitamin C, 1,000 I.U. of vitamin D3, 100 mcg of vitamin K, 100 mcg of methylcobalamin, 500 mg of magnesium, 10 mg of zinc, 1 mg of copper, 1 mg of manganese, 90 mg of glucosamine, and 3 mg of boron. The form of calcium in Bone Up is 'microcrystalline hydroxyapetite' … the actual form of calcium in bone.

My own favorite calcium supplement is 'Calcium +', manufactured by the company, Rainbow Light. The calcium in this product is in the form of a combination of an amino-acid chelate, carbonate, and citrate-malate. A serving size also provides 200 mg of vitamin C, 400 I.U. of vitamin D, 2 mg of vitamin B-6, 1000 mg of magnesium, and 1 mg of manganese; mixed in a food-source blend of 8 herbs, spirulina, and betaine. Why do I like this product ?? … it seems to agree with me metabolically, and it stops my lower leg cramps.

The following table summarizes the best non-dairy sources of calcium, in the order of most dense to least dense. I follow the same format as Table 1, and it contains several of the same food choices.

TABLE 4
Calcium Content of Selected Non-Dairy Foods
Comparison with calcium content of cow's milk

One 8 oz. cup of milk = 226 grams = 282 mg calcium

NOTE: All vegetable and legume plant foods are cooked, boiled, without salt; nuts are all dry roasted, fruits are per weight or per fruit

Food Choice	Calcium per 100 g	Calcium per cup	Amount to equal Ca content of 8 oz. milk	Amount to meet RDA of 1000 mg
Vegetables				
Tofu	201 mg	253 mg	1.1 cups	3.9 cups
Soybeans	145 mg	261 mg	1.1 cups	3.8 cups
Parsley	138 mg	83 mg	3.4 cups	12.0 cups
Turnip greens	137 mg	197 mg	1.4 cups	5.1 cups
Collards	140 mg	210 mg	1.3 cups	4.8 cups
Spinach	136 mg	245 mg	1.2 cups	4.1 cups
Watercress	120 mg	41 mg	6.9 cups	24.4 cups
Beet greens	114 mg	164 mg	1.7 cups	6.1 cups
Olives	88 mg	4 mg / olive	70.5 olives	250 olives
Taro leaves	86 mg	125 mg	2.3 cups	8.0 cups
Rhubarb	86 mg	105 mg	2.7 cups	9.5 cups
Okra	77 mg	62 mg	4.5 cups	16.1 cups
Mustard greens	74 mg	104 mg	2.7 cups	9.6 cups
Kale	72 mg	94 mg	3.0 cups	10.6 cups
Chard, Swiss	58 mg	102 mg	2.8 cups	9.8 cups
Cabbage	46 mg	36 mg	7.8 cups	27.8 cups
Celery	42 mg	63 mg	4.5 cups	15.9 cups
Broccoli	40 mg	31 mg	9.1 cups	32.3 cups
Legumes				
Cowpeas	69 mg	37 mg	7.6 cups	27.0 cups
Peanuts	55 mg	99 mg	2.8 cups	10.1 cups

Pinto beans	46 mg	79 mg	3.6 cups	12.7 cups
Snap beans	44 mg	55 mg	5.1 cups	18.2 cups
Nuts				
Almond nuts	266 mg	367 mg	0.77 cups	2.7 cups
Brazilnuts	160 mg	213 mg	1.3 cups	4.7 cups
Hazelnuts	123 mg	166 mg	1.7 cups	6.0 cups
Pistachio nuts	110 mg	135 mg	2.1 cups	7.4 cups
Pecan nuts	72 mg	97 mg	2.9 cups	10.3 cups
Macadamia nuts	70 mg	95 mg	3.0 cups	10.5 cups
Walnuts	61 mg	76 mg	3.7 cups	13.2 cups
Butternuts	53 mg	64 mg	4.4 cups	15.6 cups
Seeds				
Sesame seeds	989 mg	1,335 mg	0.2 cups	0.7 cups
Pumpkin, squash	55 mg	35 mg	8.1 cups	28.6 cups
Fruits				
Figs	162 mg	241 mg	1.2 cups	4.1 cups
Currants	86 mg	124 mg	2.3 cups	8.1 cups
Prunes	72 mg	95 mg	3.0 cups	10.5 cups
Raisins	53 mg	77 mg	3.6 cups	13.0 cups
Oranges	40 mg	52 mg / fruit	5.4 oranges	19.2 oranges
Grains				
Tortillas	175 mg	46 / tortilla	6.1 tortillas	21.7 tortillas
Bread, wheat	142 mg	36 mg / slice	7.8 slices	27.8 slices
Granola	78 mg	95 mg	2.9 cups	10.5 cups
Oat flour	55 mg	74 mg	3.8 cups	13.5 cups
Oats	54 mg	84 mg	3.4 cups	11.9 cups
Buckwheat flour	41 mg	49 mg	5.8 cups	20.4 cups
Wheat flour	34 mg	41 mg	6.9 cups	24.4 cups
Barley flour	32 mg	47 mg	6.0 cups	21.3 cups
Fish,Seafood				
Sardines	240 mg	888 mg / can	0.3 cans	1.1 cans

Anchovies	147 mg	199 mg	1.4 cups	5.0 cups
Pike	141 mg	175 mg / fillet	1.6 fillet	5.7 fillet
Ocean perch	137 mg	68 mg / fillet	4.1 fillet	14.7 fillet
Octopus	106 mg	143 mg	2.0 cups	7.0 cups
Trout	86 mg	123 mg / fillet	2.3 fillet	8.1 fillet
Halibut	60 mg	95 mg / fillet	3.0 fillet	10.5 fillet
Lobster	61 mg	88 mg	3.2 cups	11.4 cups
Crab	59 mg	79 mg / leg	3.6 legs	12.7 legs
Snapper	40 mg	68 mg / fillet	4.1 fillet	14.7 fillet
Seaweed				
Agar	625 mg	844 mg	0.3 cups	1.2 cups
Kelp	168 mg	227 mg	1.2 cups	4.4 cups
Wakame	150 mg	203 mg	1.4 cups	4.9 cups
Spirulina	120 mg	134 mg	2.1 cups	7.5 cups
Irishmoss	72 mg	97 mg	2.9 cups	10.3 cups
Egg	53 mg	26 mg / egg	10.8 eggs	38.5 eggs
Chicken	15 mg	21 mg	13.4 cups	47.6 cups
Beef	20 mg	45 mg / 8 oz	6.3 servings	22 servings
Pork	18 mg	41 mg / 8 oz	6.9 servings	24 servings

12. <u>Links with disease condition in humans</u>

The most significant link of cow's milk with disease conditions in humans is the association of the opiate molecule BCM-7, found in A1 milk, with diabetes, heart disease, schizophrenia, autism, and sudden-death syndrome. I address this issue in the next chapter, Chapter Four, the 'Ugly'.

However, there are several associations with disease separate from the BCM-7 mechanisms which can be addressed in this chapter. Various studies have identified associations with (a) allergies and allergy-related conditions, (b) breast, prostate, and stomach cancer, and (c) with heart disease.

Cancers

One fascinating study is that by Shrier et al, which actually studied the impact of lactose intolerance (lactase insufficiency) versus lactose tolerance (lactase sufficiency) on a number of disease conditions .... but the findings indirectly indicate associations with dairy intake. I reviewed this study in the section on lactose intolerance, but it warrants inclusion in this section as well. Shrier's group found that "as LNP (lactase nonpersistence) increased, stomach cancer risk increased, whereas the risks of all other conditions decreased". These other conditions were colorectal, prostate, ovarian, breast, and lung cancer, plus inflammatory bowel diseases (IBD), Crohn's disease, and ulcerative colitis ... all of which demonstrated an increased risk with lactase persistence, or lactose tolerance. (Shrier et al, 2008)

The finding that lactose intolerance was associated with an increased risk of stomach cancer makes sense ... the stress of lactose intolerance on the digestive system must have some damaging effect.

Prostate Cancer

Several studies within the last few years have found an association between dairy consumption and prostate cancer. Two notable studies are (1) *Meat and dairy consumption and subsequent risk of prostate cancer in a US cohort study*, by Rohmann et al (2007)and (2) *Dairy products, calcium and phosphorus intake, and the risk of prostate cancer: results of the French prospective SU.VI.MAX (Supplementationen Vitamines et Mineraux Antioxydants) study*, conducted by Kesse et al (2006).

Rohmann and his colleagues carried out an observation and statistical analysis study of 3,892 men 35 years of age and older who participated in the CLUE II study of Washington County, Maryland. The study was carried forward from 1989 to 2004. Their conclusion:

"Overall, consumption of processed meat, but not total meat or red meat, was associated with a possible increased risk of total prostate cancer in this prospective study. Higher intakes of dairy foods but not calcium was positively associated with prostate cancer. Further investigation into the mechanisms by which processed meat and dairy consumption might increase the risk of prostate cancer is suggested."

The Kesse et al research was another prospective study of 2,776 men over an average time span of 7.7 years. Their conclusion:

"Our data support the hypothesis that dairy products have a harmful effect with respect to the risk of prostate cancer, largely related to Ca content. The higher risk of prostate cancer with linear increasing yoghurt consumption seems to be independent of Ca and may be related to some other component."

Breast cancer

Jane Plant, in her book *Your Life In Your Hands,* presents evidence that milk consumption is one factor that can lead to breast cancer. The identified components in milk are IGF-1, as well as IGF-II and the hormone *prolatin*, which are increased when dairy cows are treated with rBGH.

Ischaemic heart disease

One researcher reviews studies that find an association of dairy consumption with ischaemic heart disease, but calls for the need for further research:

"Specific national and ethnic data suggest that a diet low or relatively low in lactose, in populations with low or relatively low prevalence of lactose absorbers, is more consistently associated with protection against ischaemic heart disease ... In seven countries with a high consumption of dairy products (six at least with a high prevalence of lactose absorbers), trends in ischaemic heart disease mortality appear to have reflected changes in the supply of milk (and therefore of lactose) ... The findings reviewed in this paper call for further investigation of the subject, epidemiologically and biochemically." (Segall, 1994)

Selected websites with negative views on cow's milk

www.all-creatures.org, this site contains a much referenced article by Michael Dye entitled *Cow's Milk is the "Perfect Food" for Baby Calves, But Many Doctors Agree it is Not Healthy for Humans*, which includes quotes by some of America's top ranking medical scientists.

www.autismweb.com, *A Parent's Guide to Autism and PDD ... the GFCF (gluten-free, casein-free) diet for autism and 'pervasive development disorder' (PDD)*

www.celiac.com, an introductory article on lactose intolerance, by Ellen Eagan.

www.dr.bretthill.com, a site sponsored by Dr. Brett Hill, a wellness expert and chiropractor

www.godairyfree.org , a daily updated site on dairy free living by Anthony Fleming

www.foodreactions.org, a site devoted to information about adverse food reactions, including lactose intolerance and cow's milk protein allergy.

www.nomilk.com, *The No Milk Page*: Books and Links, a page of many annotated links to books and sites for people wishing to avoid dairy products for health or other reasons; this is Robert Cohen's site.

www.planetlactose.blogspot.com, *The Milk-Free Bookstore and The Lactose Intolerance Clearinghouse*, compiled and maintained by Steve Carper.

www.privatehealth.co.uk, *No Cow's Milk for me Thanks*, UK's first site for lactose intolerance sufferers and the milk allergic ... useful information and bookstore.

www.tbkfitness.com, *Milk – It DOESN'T Do Your Body Good*; a well-referenced article on the association of cow's milk with heart disease, mental illness, juvenile diabetes, and prostate and testicular cancer.

Additional references for Chapter Three ... with conclusions and comments

Historical perspective

Wikipedia, *Anthropometric history,* Pertinent conclusions: "Rod Usher's *A Tall Story For Our Time* shows that one's tallness is a product of favorable living conditions ... The height of a population is, therefore, a historical record of the caloric and protein intake of the youth of that population as well as of environmental factors such as disease encounters." www.en.wikipedia.org/wiki/Anthropometric_history

Designed for cows, not for humans

Greer, F.R.; Sicherer, S.H.; Burks, A.W.; *Effects of early nutritional intervention on the development of atopic disease to infants and children: The role of maternal dietary restriction, breastfeeding, timing of introduction of complementary foods, and hydrolyzed formulas,* Pediatrics, 2008; 121: 183-91. Conclusion: Breastfeeding may delay or prevent allergies in high risk children.

New York Times, *Frank Aram Oski, 64, Retired Johns Hopkins Specialist, Dies,* December 16, 1996. An excellent summary of his life's work and contributions.

Wikipedia, *Infant Formulas,* www.en.wilipedia.org/wiki/Infant_formula A 10-page review of infant formulas and comparison with breastmilk and cow's milk. Pertinent statements: " Infant formula is nutritionally inferior to breast milk but superior to other substitutes such as animal milk. Besides breast milk, infant formula is the only other milk product which the medical community considers nutritionally acceptable for infants under the age of one year – note that solid food is nutritionally acceptable in addition to breast milk or formula during weaning.

Lactose intolerance

Campbell, A.R.; Waud, J.P.; Mathews, S. B.; *The molecular basis of lactose intolerance,* Science Progress, 2009; 92(Pt 3-4): 241-87. A review of clinical studies. Conclusion: (1) "A staggering 4,000 million people cannot digest lactose, the sugar in milk." (2) "The molecular basis of inherited hypolactasia has yet to be identified, though two polymorphisms in the introns of a helicase upstream from the lactase gene correlate closely with hypolactasis, and thus lactose intolerance." (3) "The problem of lactose intolerance has been exacerbated because of the addition of products containing lactose to various foods and drinks without being on the label."

Scrimshaw, N.S.; Murray, E.B.; *The acceptability of milk and milk products in populations with a high prevalence of lactose intolerance.* American Journal of Clinical Nutrition, Vol. 48, 1079-1159, 1988. This article is considered a classic in this field of study. Conclusions: "1) Most humans, like other mammals, gradually lose the intestinal enzyme lactase after infancy and with it the ability to digest lactose, the principle sugar in milk. At some point in prehistory, a genetic mutation occurred and lactase activity persisted in a majority of the adult population of Northern and Central Europe. 2) Persistence of intestinal lactase, the uncommon trait worldwide, is inherited as a highly penetrant autosomal-dominant characteristic. Both types of progeny are almost equally common when one parent is a lactose maldigester and the other a lactose digester. 3) The incidence of lactose maldigestion is usually determined in adults by the administration in the fasting state of a 50-g dose of lactose in water, the equivalent of that in 1 L of milk. Measurement is made of either the subsequent rise in blood glucose or the appearance of additional hydrogen in the breath. It is also sometimes identified by measuring lactase activity directly in a biopsy sample from the jejunum. For children the test dose is reduced according to weight. Depending on the severity of the lactase deficiency and other factors, the test dose may result in abdominal distention, pain, and diarrhea. 4) The frequency of lactose maldigestion varies widely among populations but is high in nearly all but those of European origin. In North American adults lactose maldigestion is found in approximately 79% of Native Americans, 75% of blacks, 51% of Hispanics, and 21% of Caucasians. In Africa, Asia, and Latin America prevalence rates range from 15-100% depending on the population studied. 5) Whenever the lactose ingested exceeds the capacity of the intestinal lactase to split it into the simple sugars glucose and galactose, which are absorbed directly, it passes undigested to the large intestine. There it is fermented by the colonic flora, with short-chain fatty acids and hydrogen gas as major products. The gas produced can cause abdominal distention and pain and diarrhea may also result from the fermentation products. 6) Among individuals with incomplete lactose digestion, there is considerable variation in awareness of lactose intolerance and in the quantity of lactose that can be ingested without symptoms. A positive standard lactose test is not a reliable predictor of the ability of an individual to consume moderate amounts of milk and milk products without symptoms. In usual situations the quantity of lactose ingested at any one time is much less than in the lactose-tolerance test."

Recommendations for dairy consumption, and political correctness

Fulgoni, V. III; Nicholis, J.; Reed, A.; Buckley, R.; Kafer, K.; Huth, P.; DiRienzo, D.; Miller, G.D.; *Dairy consumption and related nutrient intake in African-American adults and children in the United States: continuing survey of food intakes by individuals 1994 – 1996, 1998, and the National Health and Nutrition Examination Survey 1999 – 2000,* Journal of the American Dietetic Association, 2007, February; 107(2): 256-64.

Conclusion: "In this analysis, young African-American women did not meet Dietary Reference Intakes for phosphorus, and all African Americans did not meet dairy recommendations from the 2005 US Dietary Guidelines and the 2004 National Medical Association Consensus Report on the role of dairy and dairy nutrients in the diet of African Americans."

Wang, Y.; Li, S.; *Worldwide trends in dairy production and consumption and calcium intake: is promoting consumption of dairy products a sustainable solution for inadequate calcium intake?* Food Nutrition Bulletin, 2008, September; 29(3): 172-85. Conclusion: "Global production and supply of dairy products have been increasing since 1980, which has an impact on the environment. Dairy consumption and calcium intake remain low in most countries examined as compared with recommended amounts of dairy products and calcium. Promotion of consumption of dairy products does not necessarily increase total calcium intake."

Different calcium requirements for non-white ethnic groups

Lanou, A.J.; Berkow, S.E.; Barnard, N.D.; *Calcium, Dairy Products, and Bone Health in Childrent and Young Adults: A Reevaluation of the Evidence,* Pediatrics, 2005; 115; 736-743. Online version: www.pediatrics.org/cgi/content/full/115/3/736 This excellent review article supports the argument that there is a difference in calcium needs between ethnic and country populations, and that recommending dairy consumption may not be warranted: "Over the past 20 years, the National Institutes of Health, the National Academy of Sciences, and the US Department of Agriculture have made recommendations for calcium intake for children and adults for the intended purpose of osteoporosis prevention. Recommended intakes have escalated gradually, and dairy products have been promoted often in federal nutrition policy documents as a "preferred calcium source". However, because the level of dairy product consumption in the United States is among the highest in the world, accounting for 72% of dietary calcium intake, and osteoporosis and fracture rates are simultaneously high, numerous researchers have called into question the effectiveness of nutrition policies aimed at osteoporosis prevention through dairy consumption. Findings from recent epidemiological and prospective studies in women, children, and adolescents also have raised questions about the efficacy of the use of dairy products and other calcium-containing foods for the promotion of bone health. Conclusion: Scant evidence supports nutrition guidelines focused specifically on increasing milk or other dairy product intake for promoting child and adolescent bone mineralization."

Lee, W.T.; Jiang, J.; *Calcium requirements for Asian children and adolescents.* Asia Pacific Journal of Clinical Nutrition, 2008; 17 Suppl 1: 33-6. Conclusion: "Ethnic differences in calcium retention, hormonal status, bone structure, bone mineral accretion and peak bone mass are evident among Asian, Caucasian and Blacks in USA. Hence, reference calcium intakes for Asians are likely to be unique and different from those of Caucasians. More research has to be conducted in Asian populations in order to develop appropriate reference calcium intakes for the region."

Moreaboutosteoporosis.com; *All About Osteoporosis, Race or Ethnicity and Osteoporosis,* www.moreaboutosteoporosid.com/Race-or-Ethnicity-and-Osteoporosis.php Conclusion: "Studies show that Asian and Caucasian women are at highest risk for developing osteoporosis, that African-Americans have a substantially lower risk of osteoporosis and other minority populations have an intermediate risk of osteoporosis ... Instances among Native Americans are virtually unknown."

Pothiwata, P.; Evans, E.M.; Chapman-Novakofski, K.M.; *Ethnic variations in risk for osteoporosis among women: a review of biological and behavioral factors,* Journal of Women's Health, 2006, Jul-Aug; 15(6): 709-19. Conclusion: "This review summarizes evidence that white, Asian, Hispanic, and Native American women are more at risk for osteoporosis than black women ... These conclusions are supported by the disparity in BMD between white and black women ... Black women also have a lower vitamin D status than white women ... white women are more active than black and Hispanic women at all ages" What is really underscored here is that more study is needed, but that current data show marked ethnic differences in various factor relating to osteoporosis.

Walker, M.D.; Novotny, R.; Bileziklan; Weaver, C.M.; *Race and Diet Interactions in the Acqistion, Maintenance, and Loss of Bone,* Journal of Nutrition, 138" 1256S-60S, June, 2008. An observational and review study. Conclusion: "Racial differences in BMD exist and are influenced by weight, bone size, and lifestyle factors, including diet. Differences in African-Americans persist even with adjustment for these factors. Black adolescents have higher calcium retention than white adolescents across a wide range of calcium intakes, which contributes to their higher peak bone mass. Both black and white adolescents retain less calcium on high-salt diets, but the effect is more detrimental to bone in white adolescents. The response in Asians is unknown. Racial differences in fracture rates are not completely explained by differences in BMD and the role of diet is unclear. The relationship between BMD and fracture risk may be altered by racial differences in bone size, HAL (hip fracture), and bone qualities, or nonskeletal factors."

Big business in the dairy industry

Advocacy of Animals, *The Big Business of Dairy Farming: Big Trouble for Cows, www.advocacy.britannica.com/blog/advocacy/2007/06/dairy-farming* A comprehensive review of the negative aspects of big business in the dairy industry.

docstoc; *Monsanto's History of Corruption, Manipulation, and Deception,* Documents for Small Business & Professionals, This 19 page document is an excellent in-depth review of Monsanto's long history of questionable corporate productions, disposal, marketing, lobbying, and litigation, albeit quite negative. www.docstoc.com/docs/29765410

Goliath Business News, *Restructuring America's dairy farms,* The Geographical Review, January 01, 2006. An excellent, factual article reviewing the current trend in dairy farms in America, with data about Amish and other special group farms. No specific conclusion.

Nass, Meryl, MD; *Monsanto's Agent Orange: The Persistent Ghost from the Vietnam War,* Maya 12-21-2012, www.maya12-21-2012.com/2012forum/food-health/monsanto-and-agent-orange/ A factual and detailed report. Conclusion: "At a time when US tobacco corportations have been forced to pay billions of dollars in the US to compensate the victims of smoking, it would seem only reasonable that Monsanto be forced to pay billions to the Vietnamese for the catastrophe Monsanto has wrought on their country."

Organic Consumers Association, *98 Organizations Oppose Obama's Monsanto Man, Islam Siddiqui, for US Agricultural Trade Representative,* letter compiled by Dr. Marcia Ishii-Eiteman, Senior Scientist, Pesticides Action Network, and Katherine Ozer, Executive Director, National Family Farm Coalition, February 22, 2010. The conclusion is stated in the text.

Reference for Business; *Monsanto Company – Company Profile, Information, Business Description, History, Background Information on Monsanto Company,* by "Reference for Business", Company History

Index. St. Louis, Missouri, A factual report
www.referenceforbusiness.com/history2/92/Monsanto-Company.html

Source Watch, *Meat & Dairy industry,* An 11 – page review on U.S. agribusiness and its impact on trade, health and the environment. Well-referenced.
www.sourcewatch.org/index.php?itile=Meat_%25_Dairy_industry

Wikipedia, *Dairy Farming,* 2010, in-depth article on many aspects of dairy farming. No conclusion www.en.wikipedia.org/wiki/Dairy_farming

Wikipedia, *Monsanto,* www.en.wikipedia.org/wiki/Monsanto, 2010. This is an excellent 21 page review of the Monsanto Company ... including its history, corporate structure, environmental and health record, legal issues, and controversy. I have used the various Wikipedia websites extensively in my own research (Brent Bateman)

Young, Carl; *VA adds three more diseases to Agent Orange 'presumptive' list,* Times-Standard, November 18, 2009. The Department of Veteran Affairs recognizes the possible negative health effects of exposure to Agent Orange during the Vietnam War, and now extends benefits for sufferers from a total of 15 disease conditions related to Agent Orange.

Revolving Door

Edmonds Institute, *The Revolving Door,* www.edmonds-institute.org/door.html Explains the 'revolving door' concept and the Edmonds Institute's revolving door data base.

Nutrition Research Center; *Did Obama's Monsanto Choice Put the Fox in Charge of the Hen House?,* Politics of Health, July 22, 2009. www.nutritionresearchcenter.org/healthnews/did-obamas-monsanto-choice-put-the-fox-in-charge-of-the-henhouse A 6 - page expose of Michael Taylor re his appointment as senior advisor to the FDA's Administration Commissioner on Food Safety.

OEN (OpEdNews), *Monsanto and Hillary Clinton's redemptive first act as Secretary of State,* www.opednews.com/artcles/Monsanto-and-Hillary-Clint-by-Linn-Cohen-Cole-0902. Written by Linn Cohen-Cole, briefly explains the connection between the former Clinton Administration and Hillary Clinton with Monsanto and agribusiness. Makes you wonder !!

Smart Publications, *Lies and deception: How the FDA does not protect your best interests: Conflict of interest, The revolving door, The FDA and Monsanto, Bedfellows, The current situation, How Monsanto's policies have become U.S. policy,* www.smart-publications.com/nutrition/fda.php.   A well-referenced expose' of Monsanto's connections and manipulation with and within the FDA.

Spin Profiles, *Michael Taylor, "Substantial equivalence" of GM food, Bovine growth hormone, Monsanto's man Taylor returns to FDA in food-czar role, Watchdog in flack's clothing, GM and Africa, E. coli contamination,   Naotechnology   in   food   production,* www.spinprofiles.org/index.php/Michael_Taylor May 23, 2010 Includes comment by Spin Profiles, Tom Philpott, and Isabella Kenfield. This is a 12 – page expose of Michael Taylor, explaining his involvement as a government and regulator, and as a lawyer and lobbyist for Monsanto, including his invention of the "substantial equivalence" concept.

rBGH, IGF-1, anti-biotics, pesticides, and more

Bauer, K.; *New study links ADHD in kids to pesticides found on fruits and veggies,* KCBD.com   www.kcbd.com/Global/story.asp?S=12504038 Report on a recent study that showed exposure to pesticide residues on fruits and vegetables could double a child's risk of Attention Deficit Hyperactive Disorder (ADHD).

Chan, June M.; *Plasma insulin-like growth factor-1 and prostate cancer risk: a prospective study,* American Association for the Advancement of Science, Section: No. 5350, Vol. 279; Pg 563; ISSN: 0036-8075, January 23, 1998. A prospective study of 14,916 men participating in the Physicians Health Study, with follow-up over 10 years. Conclusion: "Our data support the hypothesis that higher plasma IGF-1 levels are associated with higher rates of malignancy in the prostate gland ... Finally, our results raise concern that administration of GH or IGF-1 over long periods, as proposed for elderly men to delay the effects of aging, may increase the risk of prostate cancer."

Codex Alimentarius; *Review of the Statements of Principle on the Role of Science and the Extent to which Other Factors should be Taken into Account – Application in the Case of BST and PST (Agenda Item 8),* Report of the Codex Committee on General Principles, 23rd Session www.fao.org/docrep/meeting/005/W9809E/w9809eOa.htm   This is the actual report, section 8, of the 23rd Session of Codex Alimentarius. The report is very low-key and does not come to any strong conclusions. In fact, reading the report makes one suspect that there will be a future acceptance of the U.S. position.

Cohen-Cole, Linn; *Genetically Modified Seeds: Monsanto is Putting Normal Seeds Out of Reach,* Global Researcher, April 12, 2010. The conclusion of the article is: "Monsanto contaminates the fields, trespasses onto the land taking samples and if they find any GMO plants growing there (or say they have), they then sue, saying they own the crop. It's a way to make money since farmers can't fight back in court and they settle because they have no choice. And they have done and are doing a bucket load of things to keep farmers and everyone else from having any access at all to buying, collecting, and saving of NORMAL seeds."

Epstein, Samuel S., M.D.; *What's In Your Milk, An Expose' of Industry and Government Cover-Up on the DANGERS of the Genetically Engineered (rBGH) Milk You're Drinking,* Trafford Publishing, 2006. Epstein presents a powerful expose' of the dangers of Monsanto's genetically engineered (rBGH) milk, and its no-holds-barred conspiracy to suppress this information. Dr. Epstein is professor emeritus of environmental medicine at the University of Illinois, the Chicago School of Public Health, and is Chairman of the International Cancer Prevention Coalition. He is the author of 270 scientific publications, and author or co-author of 12 books. These include the prize winning 1978 *The Politics of Cancer,* the 1995 *The Safe Shopper's Bible,* and the 2005 *Cancer-Gate: How to Win the Losing Cancer War.* He is recipient of multiple awards, including the 1998 Right Livelihood Award (the Alternative Novel Prize) for "incomparable contributions to cancer prevention, and for the leadership role in warning of the dangers of rBGH milk", the 2000 Project Censored Award (the Alternative Pulitzer Prize), and the 2005 Albert Schweitzer Golden Grand Medal "for Humanitarianism, and International Contributions to Cancer Prevention."

Fitness Uncovered, *IGF-1 (Insulin-like Growth Factor 1) in bodybuilding,* www.fitnessuncovered.co.uk Conclusion: "There is a debate between users with some who swear the hormone can be used to bring about specific site growth ... the use of IGF-1 and/or insulin can result in very serious health implications, even death."

Johansson, M.; McKay, J.D.; Wiklund, F.; Rinaldi, S.; Verheus, M.; van Gils, C.H.; Hallmans, G.; Stattin, P.; Kaacks, R.; *Implications for Prostate Cancer of Insulin-like Growth Factor-1 (IGF-1), Genetic Variation and Circulating IGF-1 Levels,* Journal of Clinical Endocrinology & Metabolism, Vol 92, No. 12: 4820-26, 2007. Conclusion: "This observation is consistent with the hypothesis that variation in the IGF-1 gene plays a role in prostate cancer susceptibility by influencing levels of IGF-1."

Larsen, H.R.; *Milk and the Cancer Connection, A comprehensive review of the evidence linking the consumption of milk from cows treated with bovine growth hormone with an increased risk of breast, prostate, and colon cancer,* International Health News, Issue 76, April 1998. This is a comprehensive review of the literature and studies prior to 1998. Conclusion: "The evidence of a strong link between cancer risk and a high level of IGF-1 is now indisputable."

Linger, Will; *U.S. and Europe Agree to Disagree on Safety of Dairy Hormone,* Press Release, June 30, 1999, by the Consumers Union, publisher of *Consumer Reports.* This is a report on the different international positions on the use and safety of rBGH and the conclusion of the 23rd Session of the U.N. Food Safety Agency, Codex Alimentarius.

Saikali, Z.; Hemani, S.; Gurmit, S.; Sujata, P.; *Role of IGF-1/IGE-1R in regulation of invasion of DU145 prostate cancer cells,* Cancer Cell International, doi: 10.2286/1475-2867-8-10, 2008 www.cancercl.com/content/   This paper summarizes clinical studies conducted at (1) Department of Research, Juravinski Cancer Center, Hamilton, Canada, (2) Department of Biochemistry and Biomedical Sciences, McMaster University, Hamilton, Canada, (3) Department of Pathology and Molecular Medicine, McMaster University, Hamilton, Canada, and (4) Department of Pediatrics, University of Alberta, Edmonton, Canada. Conclusion: "This work identifies a specific effect of IGF-1 on the invasive capacity of DU145 prostate cancer cells, and further delineates mechanisms that contribute to this effect."

Steinburg, Dan; *Monsanto's (rBGH) Genetically Modified Milk Ruled Unsafe By The UN,* Sightings, NIPCenter, www.purefood.org/rBGH/unsaferBGH.cfm, August 18, 1999. This report reviewed the conclusions of the 23rd Session of the Codex Alimentarius, plus criticized wrong interpretations of the Codex report by others.

Terry, L.C., M.D., Ph.D., Pharm.D.; *Insulin-like Growth Factor-1 (IGF-1, Somatomedin C) Blood Levels Are Not Associated With Prostate Specific Antigen (PSA) Levels or Prostate Cancer: A Study fo 749 patients,* Medical College of Wisconsin, Milwaukee, www.thehormoneshop.com/prostate.htm

Tokar, Brian; *Monsanto, A Checkered History,* Mindfully.org, www.mindfully.org/Industry/Monsanto-Checkered-HistoryOct98.htm Another expose' of the Monsanto Company.

Warwick, Hugh; *Agent Orange: The Poisoning of Vietnam,* The Ecologist, Vol 28, No. 5, Sept/Oct, 1998. Warwicks conclusion: "Monsanto was heavily involved in, and was the major financial beneficiary of one of the most shocking scandals of our age."

Wikipedia, *Bovine Somatotropin,* Wikipedia, The Free Encyclopedia, www.en.wikipedia.org/Bovine_somatotropin, 2010. This is an excellent online source, factual and objective.

Wolk, A.; Mantzoros, C.S.; Anderson, S.O.; Bergstrom, R.; Signorello, L.B.; Lagiou, P.; Adami, H.O.; Trichopoulos, D.; *Insulin-like growth factor 1 and prostate cancer risk: a population-based, case-control study.* Journal of the National Cancer Institute, June 17, 90(12): 911-5, 1998. A clinical study of 210 patients and 224 controls in Sweden, with statistical analysis. Conclusion: "Elevated serum IGF-1 levels may be an important predictor of risk for prostate cancer."

Blood, pus, and manure

Bradley, A.; Green, M.; *Use and Interpretation of somatic cell count data in dairy cows.* In Practice, 27: 310-15, 2005. Conclusion: "Although a raised SCC is an accepted indicator of an existing bacterial infection, a very low SCC has been associated with an increased subsequent susceptibility to clinical mastitis. This suggests that somatic cells may provide protection from bacterial colonization as well as being a marker of infection."

Pennington, J.A.; *Reducing Somatic Cell Count in Dairy Cattle,* Cooperative Extension Service, University of Arkansas, www.uaex.edu 2010. A guide to dairy farmers on how to reduce the somatic cell count in their milk.

Smith, K.L.; *A Look at Physiological and Regulatory SCC Standards in Milk,* NMC Newsletter, "Udder Topics", December, 1997. Excerpted from a paper presented by K. Larry Smith, Ohio State University, at the International Dairy Federation (IDF) meeting in Vienna, Austria, September, 1995. This article is an excellent overview of what is known about SCC and mastitis. Conclusion: "These data argue in favor of the European Union SCC standard of 400,000 as the basis of international trade in safe, high quality, milk and milk products."

Tschang, Chi-Chu; *Milk Contamination Is Sinking China's Farmers,* Bloomberg Businessweek, October 2, 2008. This article highlights the current problem that China is experiencing with milk contamination.

Labeling requirements

Consumer Reports, July, 2008; *Any Artificial Hormones?*, an update on Monsanto's lobbying campaign to keep "rBGH–free" off of milk labels. Monsanto responded with their own report entitled *Consumer's Reports' Errors of Milk Labeling,* , claiming that the description of their efforts was completely inaccurate, reciting as fact that (a) the use of rBGH has no adverse effect on the animals, and (b) that there is no difference in milk from cows supplemented with Posilac and milk from cows that have not received Prosilac.
www.monsanto.com/monsant_today/for_the_record/consumer_reports_milk_labeling

Scott-Thomas; *Senators propose country of origin labeling for dairy,* Food Navigator, October 20, 2009. www.foodnavigator-usa.com/Legislation/Senators-propose-country-of-origin-labeling. Senators Brown (D-OH), Fiengold (D-WI), and Franken (D-MN) have introduced a bill requiring coutry-of-origin-labeling (COOL) on all dairy products.

Milk, calcium, protein, and osteoporosis ... a possible paradox

Fogarty, P.; O'Beirne, B.; Casery, C.; *Epidemiology of the most frequent diseases in the European a-symptomatic post-menopausal women: Is there any difference between Ireland and the rest of Europe?,* Maturitas, 2005, November 15; Vol. 52, Supplement 1, Pages 3-6. Conclusion: "There is a marked European geographic distribution of osteoporosis. Rates are higher in Scandinavia than in the Southern European countries. The possible reasons for this higher incidence of osteoporotic fractures in the Northern European countries is associated with the climate, which limits physical activity and exposure to sunlight and increases the risk of falls."

Qaseem, A.; Snow, V.; Shekelle, P.; Hopkins, R.; Forciea, M.A.; Owens, D.K.; *Screening for Osteoporosis in Men: A Clinical Practic Guideling from the American College of Physicians,* Clinical Guideline, American College of Physicians, Annual Internal Medicine, 2008; 148: 680-84. Conclusion: "High-quality evidence show that age, low body weight, physical exercise, and weight loss are strong predictors of an increased risk for osteoporosis in men. There is also moderate-quality evidence that previous fragility fracture, systemic corticosteroid therapy, androgen deprivation therapy, and spinal cord injury are predictors of an increased risk for osteoporosis in men. Cigarette smoking and low dietary intake of calcium predict low bone mass."

Ralston, S.H.; *Genetics of osteoporosis,* Annals of the New York Academy of Sciences, 2010, March; 1192(1): 181-9. Conclusion: "Osteoporosis is a common disease with a strong genetic component ... Twin and family studies have shown that the heritability of bone mineral density and other determinants of fracture risk, such as ultrasound properties of bone, skeletal geometry, and bone turnover, is high, although heritability of fracture is modest. Many different genetic variants contribute to the regulation of these phenotypes. Most are common variants of small effect size, but there is evidence that rare variants of large effect size also contribute in some individuals. Many of the genes that regulate susceptibility to osteoporosis have been identified through studies of rare bone diseases, but genome-wide association studies have also been successful in identifying genes that predispose to osteoporosis."

Sadat-Ali, M.; AlElq, A.; *Osteoporosis among male Saudi Arabs: A pilot study,* Annals of Saudi Medicine, 2006; 26: 450-4. A prospective study of 115 males 50 – 76 years of age. Conclusion: "Our study indicates that the prevalence of osteoporosis among Saudi Arabian males is higher than among Western males."

Tsugawa, N.; *Vitamin D and osteoporosis: current topics from epidemiological studies,* Rinsho Byori / The Japanese Journal of Clinical Pathology, 2010, March; 58(3): 244-53 Conclusion: "Increases of fracture of bedridden and mortality rates associated with facture are serious social problems in Japan ... It is known that a mild decrease in the serum 25-D concentration (vitamin D insufficiency) leads to secondary hyperparathyroidism, which has a negative effect on bone metabolism in the elderly. Therefore, vitamin D insufficiency is thought to be one of the risk factors for osteoporosis. Vitamin D insufficiency is common throughout the world. In Japan, we have also confirmed that around half of elderly women show vitamin D insufficiency."

Uenishi, K.; *Nutrition and bone health. Present knowledge and practice,* Clinical Calcium, 2009, July; 19(7): 1028-31. Expert statement: "All the components which constitute our body are reconstructed from the nutrients taken in from foods. Bone is also the same and various nutrients are involved for the formation and maintenance: calcium, vitamin D, protein, vitamin K, magnesium, zinc, vitamin B group, vitamin A, etc."

Osteoporosis ... lack of statistics

Lau, E.M.; Lee, J.K.; Suriwongpaisal, P. Saw, S.M.; Das De, S.; Khir, A.; Sambrook, P.; *The incidence of hip fractures in four Asian countries: the Asian Osteoporosis Study (AOS),* Osteoporosis International, 2001; 12(3): 239-43. This was the first study of its kind done. Only the number of persons over 50 who were discharged from hospitals with a diagnosed hip fracture was enumerated, showing a low incidence of osteoporosis. Conclusion: "We conclude that there is moderate variation in the incidence of hip fractures among Asian countries. The rates were highest in urbanized countries. With rapid economic development in Asia, hip fractures will prove to be a major public health challenge."

Woolf, A.D.; Pfleger, B.; *Burden of osteoporosis and fractures in developing countries,* Current Osteoporosis Reports, Current Medidine Group LLC, Vol. 3, Number 3 / September, 2005. Conclusion: " The burden of osteoporosis in developing countries is increasing dramatically with the aging of the population and demographic trends; however, there is a lack of direct epidemiological date. There are clear differences at present between and within populations that limits the validity of may estimates and more data is needed."

Osteoporosis ... possible confounders ... vitamin D, latitude and sunlight, and skin-coloring

Linus Pauling Institue, *Vitamin D,* Linus Pauling Institute at Oregon State University. This is an in-depth review of studies on vitamin D and conclusions. Regarding osteoporosis, the conclusions include: (1) "In vitamin D deficiency, calcium absorption cannot be increased enough to satisfy the body's calcium nees. Consequently, PTH production by the parathyroid glands is increased and calcium is mobilized from the skeleton to maintain normal serum calcium levels – a condition known as secondary *hyperparathyroidism*." (2) "Although osteoporosis is a multifactorial disease, vitamin D insufficiency can be an important contributing factor ... Without sufficient vitamin D from sun exposure or dietary intake, intestinal calcium absorption cannot be maximized

148

...Solar ultraviolet-B-radiation (UVB; wavelengths of 290 to 315 nanometers). People with dark –colored skin synthesize markedly less vitamin D on exposure to sunlight than those with light-colored skin. Additionaly, the elderly have diminished capacity to synthesize vitamin D from sunlight exposure and frequently use sunscreen or protective clothing in order to prevent skin cancer and skin damage. In latitudes around 40 degrees north or 40 degrees south (Boston is 42 degrees north), there is insufficient UVB radiation available for vitamin D synthesis from November to early March. Ten degrees farther north or south (Edmonton, Canada) the "vitamin D winter" extends from mid-October to Mid-March ... Vitamin D toxicity (hypervitaminosis D) induces abnormally high serum calcium levels (hypercalcemia), which could result in bone loss, kidney stones, and calcification of organs like the heart and kidneys if untreated over a long period of time."

Osteoporosis ... other factors

Bass, S.L.; Naughton, G.; Saxon, L.; Iuliano-Burns, S.; Daly, R.; Briganti, E.M.; Hume, C.; Howson, C.; *Exercise and calcium combined results in a greater osteogenic effect than either factor alone: a blinded randomized placebo-controlled trial in boys,* Journal of Bone and Mineral Research, 2007, March; 22(3): 458-64. A blinded, randomized, placebo-controlled study of 88 pre- and early-puberty boys. Conclusion: "In this group of normally active boys with adequate calcium intakes, additional exercise and calcium supplementation resulted in a 2-3% greater increase in BMC than controls at the loaded sites. These findings strengthen the evidence base for public health campaigns to address both exercise and dietary changes in children for optimizing the attainment of peak BMC."

Budak, N.; Cicek, B.; Sahin, H. Tutus, A.; *Bone mineral density and serum 25-hydroxyvitamin D level: is there any difference according to the dressing style of the female university students,* International Journal of Food Sciences and Nutrition, 2004, November; 55(7): 569-75. An observation study of 67 female students divided by dress styles. The finding was that a dress style that covered all of the body except the face and hands was associated with a lower vitamin D status and lower BMD.

High protein intakes cause bone loss

Bonjour, J.P.; *Dietary protein: an essential nutrient for bone health,* Journal of the American College of Nutrition, 2005, December: 24(6 Suppl): 526S-36S. Conclusion: "Consequently, dietary proteins are as essential as calcium and vitamin D for bone health and osteoporosis prevention. Furthermore, there is no consistent evidence of superiority of vegetal over animal proteins on calcium metabolism, bone loss prevention and risk reduction of fragility fractures."

Heaney, R.P.; Layman, D.K.; *Amount and type of protein influences bone health,* American Journal of Clinical Nutrition, 2008, May; 87(5): 1567S-1578S. Conclusion: "Intakes of both calcium and protein must be adequate to fully realize the benefit of each nutrient on bone. Optimal protein intake for bone health is likely higher than current recommended intakes, particularly in the elderly. Concerns about dietary protein increasing urinary calcium appear to be offset by increases in absorption. Likewise, concerns about the impact of protein on acid production appear to be minor compared with the alkalinizing effects of fruits and vegetables."

Misra,D.; Berry, S.D.; Broe, K.E.; McLean, R.R.; Cupples, L.A.; Tucker, K.L.; Kiel, D.P.; Hannan, M.T.; *Does dietary protein reduce hip fracture risk in elders? The Framingham osteoporosis study,* Osteoporosis International, May 5, 2010. Conclusion: "Our results are consistent with reduced risk of hip fracture with higher dietary protein intake." The results of this study directly contradicts the statements by McDougall and others that high protein consumption is a cause of osteoporosis.

The acid-base imbalance hypothesis

Bruckhardt, P.; *Mineral waters and bone health,* Revue Medicale de la Suisse Romande, 2004, February: 124(2): 101-3. Conclusion: "Some mineral waters contain minerals in such high concentration that they can influence bone health when consumed regularly. Calcium from mineral water is readily absorbed, inhibits PTH secretion and bone resorption on the short as well as on the long term. Sodium concentrations are too low to bother, sulfates have no documented bone effect, but fluoride can in rare cases be so high that it increases bone density. Since potassium and bicarbonate lower renal calcium excretion, and since the latter improves calcium balance, mineral waters rich in bicarbonate and potassium have been tested. Indeed, they lowered renal excretion and bone resorption in short and medium term trials, and they could be of particular interest in the prevention of osteoporosis in addition to calcium-rich waters."

Fenton, T.R.; Eliasziw, M.; Tough, S.C.; Lyon, A.W.; Brown, J.P.; Hanley, D.A.; *Low urine pH and acid excretion do not predict bone fractures of the loss of bone mineral density: a prospective cohort study,* BMC Musculoskeletal Disorders, May 10, 2010; 11(1): 88. This was a prospective cohort study of the 651 subjects in the Canadian Multicentre Osteoporosis Study. Conclusion: "The alkaline diet and related products are marketed to the general public. Websites, lay literature, and direct mail marketing encourage people to measure their urine pH to assess their health status and their risk of osteoporosis. CONCLUSION: Urine pH and urine acid excretion do not predict osteoporosis risk."

Fenton, T.R.; Lyon, A.W.; Eliasziw, M.; Tough, S.C.; Hanley, D.A.; *Phosphate decreases urine calcium and increases calcium balance: a meta-analysis of the osteoporosis acid-ash diet hypothesis,* Nutrition Journal, 2009, September; 15;8:41. This is a second study by Fenton et al which discredits the acid-ash diet hypothesis. The introduction states: "The acid-ash hypothesis posits that increased excretion of 'acidic' ions derived from the diet, such as phosphate, contributes to net acidic ion excretion, urine calcium excretion, demineralization of bone, and osteoporosis. The public is advised by various media to follow an alkaline diet to lower their acidic ion intakes. The objectives of this meta-analysis were to quantify the contribution of phosphate to bone loss in healthy adult subjects." This study could be considered a landmark contribution. Their abstract outlines their methods, results, and conclusions: " Methods: Literature was identified through computerized searches regarding phosphate with surrogate and/or direct markers of bone health, and was assessed for methodological quality. Multiple linear regression analyses, weighted for sample size, were used to combine the study results. Tests of interaction included stratification by calcium intake and degree of protonation of the phosphate supplement. Results: Twelve studies including 30 intervention arms manipulated 269 subjects' phosphate intakes. Three studies reported net acid excretion. All of the meta-analyses demonstrated significant decreases in urine calcium excretion in response to phosphate supplements whether the calcium intake was high or low, regardless of the degree of protonation of the phosphate supplement. None of the meta-analyses revealed lower calcium balance in response to increased phosphate intakes, whether the calcium intake was high or low, or the composition of the phosphate supplement. Conclusion: All of the findings from this meta-analysis were contrary to the acid ash hypothesis. Higher phosphate intakes

151

were associated with decreased urine calcium and increased calcium retention. This meta-analysis did not find evidence that phosphate intake contributes to demineralization of bone or to bone calcium excretion in the urine. Dietary advice that dairy products, meats, and grains are detrimental to bone health due to "acidic" phosphate content needs reassessment. There is no evidence that higher phosphate intakes are detrimental to bone health.

Ishimi, Y.; *Nutrition and bone health. Magnesium and Bone,* Clinical Calcium, 2010, May; 20(5): 762-7. Conclusion: "Maganesium is one of the essential minerals for bone formation. In the magnesium-deficient rats, apparent bone loss caused by increase in bone resorption and decrease in bone formation was observed. Although epidemiological studies suggest that magnesium deficiency is one of the risk factors for osteoporosis, a relationship between magnesium intake and bone mineral density is not clear."

Jojoo, R.; Song, L.; Rasmussen, H.; Harris, S.S.; Dawson-Hughes, B.; *Dietary Acid-Base Balance, Bone Resorption, and Calcium Excretion,* Journal of the American College of Nutrition, Vol. 25, No. 3, 224-230. A diet-intervention study of 40 healthy older men on special diets for 60 days. Conclusion: "Diet changes that increase renal NAE as associated with increases in serum PTH, bone resorption, and calcium excretion over a 60-day period.

Macdonald, H.M.; New, S.A.; Fraser, W.D.; Campbell, M.K.; Reid, D.M.; *Low dietary potassium intakes and high dietary estimates of net endogenous acid production are associated with low bone mineral density in premenopausal women and increased markers of bone resorption in postmenopausal women,* American Journal of Clinical Nutrition, 2005, April; 81(4): 923-33. Conclusion: "Dietary potassium, an indicator of NEAP (net endogenous acid production) and fruit and vegetable intake, may exert a modest influence on markers of bone health, which over a lifetime may contribute to a decreased risk of osteoporosis.

Marangella, M.; Di Stefano, M.; Casalis, S.; Berutti, S.; D'Amelio, P.; Isaia, G.C.; *Effects of potassium citrate supplementation on bone metabolism,* Calcified Tissue International, 2004, April; 74(4): 330-5. Conclusion: "Our results suggest that treatment with an alkaline salt, such as potassium citrate, can reduce bone resorption thereby contrasting the potential adverse effects caused by chonic academia of protein-rich diets.

McGartland, C.P.; Robson, P.J.; Murray, L.J.; Cran, G.W.; Savage, M.J.; Watrkins, D.C.; Rooney, M.M., Boreham, C.A.; *Fruit and vegetable consumption and bone mineral density: the Northern Ireland Young Hearts Project,* American Journal of Clinical Nutrition, 2004, October; 80(4): 1019-23. Conclusion: "High intakes of fruit may be important for bone health in girls. It is possible that fruit's alkaline-forming properties mediate the body's acid-base balance. However, intervention studies are required to confirm the findings of observational study."

Two excellent factual articles explaining the acid-base concept from a medical point of view. Regarding calcium loss, there is no normal role of calcium used in the 3 acid-base homeostasis functions, which operate either via the respiratory system, the kidneys, or the buffer system.

Remer, T; *Influence of nutrition on acid-base balance – metabolic aspects,* European Journal of Nutrition, 2001, October: 40(5): 214-20. In 1995 Remer calculated the renal net acid excretion (NAE) and is responsible for the derivation of the 'potential renal acid load' (PRAL) of foods. He is frequently referenced by writers from the vegetarian camp. In this light, his abstract conclusion is of particular interest: "An adequate concept to estimate renal NAE and potential renal acid loads from dietary intakes must consider the specific bioabavailability of the individual nutrients. Furthermore, an increased protein intake does not necessarily result in a accordingly increased use of endogenous acid excretion capacity for two reasons: (1) additional alkali loads in an appropriately composed diet can compensate for the protein-related raised acid production and (2) protein itself moderately improves the renal capacity to excrete net acid by increasing the endogenous supply of ammonia which is the major urinary hydrogen ion acceptor."

Remer, T.; Dimitriou, T., Manz, F.; *Dietary potential renal acid load and renal ne acid excretion in healthy, free-living children and adolescents,* American Journal of Clinical Nutrition, 2003, May; 77(5): 1255-60. A clinical analysis study of 165 children and 73 adoloescents. Conclusion: "Predicting NAE from dietary intakes, food tables, and anthropometric data is also applicable during growth and yields appropriate estimates even when self-selected diets are consumed. The PRAL estimate based on only 4 nutrients (protein, phosphorus, potassium, and magnesium) may allow relatively simple assessments of the acidity of foods and diets."

Tucker, K.L.; *Dietary intake and bone status with aging,* Current Pharmaceutical Design, 2003; 9(32): 2687-704. Expert statement: "...

most of the attention to dietary risk factors for osteoporosis has focused almost exclusively on calcium and vitamin D. Recently, there has been considerable interest in the effects of a variety of other nutrients on bone status. These include minerals – magnesium, potassium, copper, zinc, silicon, sodium; vitamins – vitamin C, vitamin K, vitamin B-12, vitamin A; and macronutrients – protein, fatty acids, sugars. In addition, foods and food components, including milk, fruit and vegetables, soy products, carbonated beverages, mineral water, dietary fiber, alcohol and caffeine have recently been examined. Together the evidence clearly suggests that prevention of bone loss through diet is complex and involves many nutrients and other food constituents."

Calcium and weight control

Barba, G.; Russo, P.; *Dairy foods, dietary calcium and obesity: a short review of the evidence,* Nutrition, Metabolism & Cardiovascular Diseases, 2006, September; 16(6): 445-51. A review of data from cross-sectional epidemiological studies compared with prospective and randomized controlled intervention trials. Conclusion: "Available data do not unequivocally support the hypothesis that a causal relationship exists between high dairy food intake--and/or high dietary calcium intake—and lower fat mass deposition."

Barr, S.I.; *Increased dairy product or calcium intake: is body weight or composition affected in humans?,* Journal of Nutrition, 2003, January; 133(1): 245S-48S. A review of MEDLINE studies. Conclusion: "The data available from randomized trials of dairy products or calcium supplementation provide little support for an effect in reducing body weight or fat mass."

Florito, I.M.; Ventura, A.K.; Mitchell, D.C.; Smiciklas-Wright, H.; Birch, L.L.; *Girls' dairy intake, energy intake, and weight status,* Journal of the American Dietetic Association, 2006, November; 106(11): 1851-6. A cross-sectional study of 172 11-year-old non-Hispanic white girls. Conclusion: "Our findings reveal that reporting bias, resulting from the presence of a substantial proportion of underreporters of higher weight status, can contribute to obtaining spurious associations between dairy intake and weight status."

Harvey-Berino, J.; Gold, J.; Lauber, R.; Starinski, A.; *The Impact of calcium and dairy product consumption on weight loss,* Obesity Research, 2005, October: 13(10): 1720-6. Intervention study of 54 subjects for 12 months. Conclusion: "These findings suggest that a high-dairy calcium diet does not substantially improve weight loss beyond what can be achieved in a behavioral intervention."

Lanou, A.J.; Barnard, N.D.; *Dairy and weight loss hypothesis: an evaluation of the clinical trials,* Nutrition Reviews, 2008, May; 66(5): 272-9. A review of 49 randomized trials assessing the effect of dairy productrs or calcium supplementation on body weight. Conclusion: "41 showed no effect, two demonstrated weight gain, one showed a lower rate of gain, and five showed weight loss. Consequently, the majority of the current evidence from clinical trials does not support the hypothesis that calcium or dairy consumption aids in weight or fat loss."

Lorenzen, J.K.; Molgaard, C.; Michaelsen, K.F.; Astrup, A.; *Calcium supplementation for 1 yr. does not reduce body weight or fat mass in young girls.* American Journal of Clinical Nutrition, 2006, January; 83(1): 18-23. A randomized, double-blind, placebo-controlled intervention study of 110 young girls. Conclusion: "Habitual dietary calcium intake was inversely associated with body fat, but a low-dose calcium supplement had no effect on body weight, height, or body fat over 1 year in young girls."

Phillips, S.M.; Bandini, L.G.; Cyr, H.; Colclough-Douglas, S.; Naumova, E.; Must, A.; *Dairy food consumption and body weight and fatness studied longitudinally over the adolescent period,* International Journal of Obesity and Related Metabolic Disorders, 2003, September; 27(9): 1106-13. A longitudinal study of 196 girls from the MIT Growth and Development Study. Conclusion: "We find no evidence that dairy food consumption is associated with BMI z-score or %BF (percent body-fat) during adolescence."

Snijder, M.B.; van der Heijden, A.A.; van Dam, R.M.; Stehouwer, C.D.; Hiddink, G.J.; Nijpels, G.; heine, R.J.; *Is higher dairy consumption associated with low body weight and fewer metabolic disturbances? The Hoorn Study,* American Journal of Clinical Nutrition, 2007, April; 85(4): 989-95. Cross-sectional study of 2064 Dutch men and women aged 50-75 years. Conclusion: "In an elderly Dutch population, higher dairy consumption was not associated with lower weight or more favorable levels of components of the metabolic syndrome, except for a modest association with lower blood pressure."

Weker, H.; *Simple obesity in children. A study on the role of nutritional factors.* Medycyna wieku rozwojowego, 2006, Jan-Mar; 10(1): 3-191. A Polish observation study of 236 children. Conclusion: "The main risk factors for simple obesity were familial and environmental conditions." However, the authors recognized that "significant body mass loss has been observed in children in whose diet the amount of proteins and their share of the total energy value only slightly differs from the level before the dietary treatment."

Calcium, dairy, and bone

Iuliano-Burns, S.; Wang, X.F.; Evans, A.; Bonjour, J.P. Seeman, E.; *Skeletal benefits from calcium supplementation are limited in children with calcium intakes near 800 mg daily,* Osteoporosis International, 2006, December; 17(12): 1794-800. An intervention study of 99 boys and girls aged 5-11 years who were supplemented for 12 months. Conclusion: "In healthy children consuming about 800 mg calcium daily, calcium supplementation with milk minerals of calcium carbonate does not appear to produce biologically meaningful benefits to skeletal health."

Konstantynowicz, J.; Nguyen, T.V.; Kaczmarski, M.; Jamiolkowski, J.; Piotrowska-Jastrzebska, J.; Seeman, E.; *Fractures during growth: potential role of a milk-free diet,* Osteoporosis International, 2007, December; 18(12): 1601-7 A case-controlled study of 57 boys and 34 girls in Poland, aged 2.5 – 20 years with fractures randomly matched with 171 boys and 102 girls without fractures. Conclusion: "These data suggest that the contribution of milk-free-diet to fracture liability among children and adolescents is modest."

Lanou, A.J.; Berkow, S.E.; Barnard, N.D.; *Calcium, dairy products, and bone health in children and young adults; a reevaluation of the evidence,* Pediatrics, 2005, March; 115(3): 736-43. A review of 58 studies, which included 22 cross-sectional studies, 13 retrospective studies, 10 longitudinal prospective studies, and 13 randomized, controlled trials. Conclusion: "Scant evidence supports nutrition guidelines focused specifically on increasing milk or other dairy product intake for promoting child and adolescent bone mineralization."

Calcium and hypertension

Karppanen, H.; Karpanen, P.; Mervaala, E.; *Why and how to implement sodium, potassium, calcium, and magnesium changes in food items and diets?* Journal of Human Hypertension, 2005, December; 19 Suppl 3: S10-9. An expert statement. Summary: "Decreased intakes of sodium alone, and increased intakes of potassium, calcium, and magnesium each alone decrease elevated blood pressure ... the present average potassium, calcium, and magnesium intakes are remarkably lower than the recommended intake levels (DRI). In the USA, for example, the average intake of these minerals is only 35-50% of the recommended intakes ... The present average sodium intakes, approximately 3000 – 4500 mg/day in various industrialized populations, are very high. There is convincing evidence which indicates that this imbalance, that is, the high intake of sodium on one hand and the low intakes of potassium, calcium, and magnesium on the other hand, produce and maintain elevated blood pressure in a big proportion of the population." This suggests that, contrary to the dairy/low pressure hypothesis, that it is not only calcium that affects lowered blood pressure, and that perhaps the low sodium content of dairy is a factor. Note that milk is very low in magnesium and potassium.

Cancer

Genkinger, J.M.; Hunter, D.J.; Spiegelman, D.; Anderson, K.E.; Arsian, A.; Beeson, W.L.; Buring, J.E.; Fraser, G.E.; Freudenheim, J.L.; Goldbohm, R.A.; Hankinson, S.E.; Jacobs, D.R. Jr.; Koushik, A.; Lacey, J.V. Jr.; Larsson, S.C.; Leitzmann, M.; McCullough, M.L.; Miller, A.B.; Rodriguez, C.; Rohan, T.E.; Schouten, L.J.; Shore, R.; Smit, E.; Wolk, A.; Zhang, S.M.; Smith-Warner, S.A.; *Dairy products and ovarian cancer: a pooled analysis of 12 cohort studies.* Cancer Epidemiology, Biomarkers & Prevention, 2006, February; 15(2): 364-72 A meta-analysis study of 14 cohort studies. Conclusion: "A modest elevation in the risk of ovarian cancer was seen for lactose intake at the level that was equivalent to three or more servings of milk per day."

Diabetes

Dahl-Jergensen, K.; Joner, G.; Hanssen, K.F.; *Relationship between cow's milk consumption and incidence of IDDM in childhood.* Diabetes Care, 1991, November; 14(11): 1081-3 Incidence rates of diabetes in children 0-14 years. An ecological correlation study. Incidence rates validated by the Diabetes Epidemiology Research International Study Group from Finland, Sweden, Norway, Great Britain, Denmark, United States, New Zealand, Netherlands, Canada, France, Israel, and Japan were used. Conclusion: "Correlation between milk consumption and incidence of insulin-dependent diabetes mellitus (IDDM) was r = 0.96.

The results support the hypothesis that cow's milk may contain a triggering factor of the development of IDDM."

Virtanen, Hypponen, E.; S.M.; Laara, E.; Vahasalo, P.; Kulmala, P.; Savola, K.; Rasanen, L.; Aro, A.; Knip, M.; Akerblom, H.K.; *Cow's milk consumption, disease-associated autoantibodies and type 1 diabetes mellitus: a follow-up study in siblings of diabetic children Childhood Diabetes in Finland Study Group.* Diabetic Medical Journal, 1998, September: 15(9): 730-8 Conclusion: "This study suggests that high consumption of cow's milk during childhood may be associated both with seroconversion to positivity for diabetes-associated autoantibodies and progression to clinical Type 1 diabetes mellitus among siblings of children with diabetes."

Virtanen, S.M.; Laara, E.; Hypponen, E.; Reijonen, H.; Rasanen, L.; Aro, A.; Knip, M.; Ilonen, J.; Akerblom, H.K.; *Cow's milk consumption, HLA-DQB1 genotype, and type 1 diabetes: a nested case-control study of siblings of children with diabetes. Childhook diabetes in Finland study group.* Diabetes, 2000, June; 49(6): 912-7 Conclusion: "Our results provide support for the hypothesis that high consumption of cow's milk during childhood can be diabetogenic in siblings of children with type 1 diabetes."

Dairy products, calcium ... and hypertension

Engberink, M.F.; Geleijinse, J.M.; de Jong, N.; Smit, H.A.; Kok, F.J.; Verschuren, W.M.; *Dairy intake, blood pressure, and incident hypertension in a general Dutch population,* Journal of Nutrition, 2009, March; 139(3): 582-7. An observational study observing the relation of dairy intake with blood pressure in 21,553 Dutch participants aged 20-65 years. Conclusion: "We conclude that variations in BP in a general middle-aged Dutch population cannot be explained by overall dairy intakes."

Fertility

Cramer, D.W.; Huijuan, X.; Sahi, T.; *Adult Hyupolactasia, Milk Consumption, and Age-specific Fertility.* American Journal of Epidemiology, 1994, Vol. 139, No. 3: 282-89. An epidemiological correlation study. Conclusion: "The authors found significant correlations among these variables such that fertility at older ages is lower and the decline in fertility with aging is steeper in populations with high per capita consumption of milk and greater ability to digest its lactose."

Infectious disease

Atkins, P.J.; *White Poison? The Social Consequences of Milk Consumption, 1850-1930,* Social History of Medicine, 1992; 5(2): 207-227. Historical research. Conclusion: "Local authority regulation and central government legislation were very slow in controlling the cleanliness of production and sale. Milk was heavily contaminated with bacteria and was responsible for spreading a variety of diseases such as scarlet fever and tuberculosis. Infants not wholly breastfed were particularly vulnerable to diarrhoeal infections. Improvements such as pasteurization and bottling were slow to spread and are unlikely to have had much impact before the 1920's. Overall it is argued that ill-health caused by dirty milk was more serious , and its amelioration much later than previously documented."

Heart Disease

Lorenz, M.; Jochmann, N.; von Krosigk, A.; Martus, P.; Baumann, G.; Stangl, V.; *Addition of milk prevents vascular protective effects of tea.* European Heart Journal, 2007, January; 28(2): 219-23   A clinical analysis study with 16 healthy female volunteers. Conclusion: "Milk counteracts the favourable health effects of tea on vascular function."

Houston, D.K.; Driver, K.E.; Bush, A.J.; Kritchevsky, S.B.; *The association between cheese consumption and cardiovascular risk factors among adults,* Journat of Human Nutrition and Dietetics, 2008, April; 21(2): 129-40   Analysis study from NHANES III data (10,872 subjects). Conclusion: "More frequent cheese consumption was associated with less favorable body composition and cardiovascular risk profile in men."

Triolo, G.; Accardo-Palumbo, A.; Dieli, F.; Ciccia, F.; Ferrante, A.; Giardina, E.; Licata, G.; *Humoral and cell mediated immune response to cow's milk proteins in Behcet's disease,* Annals of the Rheumatic Diseases, 2002, May; 61(5): 459-62   Clincal study on 46 patients with Behcet's disease and 37 healthy controls. Conclusion: "The results indicate that an active immune response occurs in Behcet's disease. This response involves an increased frequency of antibodies to cow's milk protein and a strong Th1 polarization after exposure to these antigens. The occurrence of these abnormalities supports a putative role for cow's milk proteins immune response in the pathogenesis of Behcet's disease."   Behcet's disease is a form of vasulitis (disease of the vascular system) that can lead to arterial ulceration and lesions, and is thought to be the result of a chronic disturbance in the body's immune system.

Stroke

Larsson, S.C.; Mannisto, S.; Virtanen, M.J.; Konito, J.; Albanes, D.; Virtamo, J.; *Dairy foods and risk of stroke,* Epidemiology, 2009, May; 20(3): 355-60. Data analysis from the Alpha-Tocopherol, Beta-Carotene Cancer Prevention Study. Conclusion: "These findings suggest that the intake of certain dairy foods may be associated with risk of stroke."

References used in the text for Chapter Three

AAFP, American Academy of Family Physicians, *Breastfeeding (Policy Statement* (1989) (2007) www.aafp.org/online/en/home/policy

AAP, American Academy of Pediatrics, *Policy Statement: Breastfeeding and the Use of Human Milk;* Pediatrics, Vol. 115, No.2. February 2005: pp 496-506

AFN, *Nocton's 'giant dairy' plan scuttled in UK,* an article by Katy Humphries, Just-Food, www.ausfoodnews.com.au;2010/04/15/noctons-giant-dairy-plan-scuttled-in-uk.html , April 15, 2010

Arnaud, C.D.; Sanchez, S.D.; *Calcium and Phosphorus,* Chapter 24 of *Present Knowledge in Nutrition, Seventh Edition,* Edited by E.E. Ziegler and L.J. Filer, Jr., International Life Sciences Institute, 1996.

Atkins, P.J.; White Poison? The Social Consequences of Milk Consumption, 1850-1930, Social History of Medicine, 1992; 5(2): 207-227.

Berardi, J.M.; *Covering Nutritional Bases, The Importance fo Acid-Base Balance,* Johnberardi.com July 13, 2003

Berton, P.; Barnard, N.D.; Mills, M.; *Racial bias in federal nutrition policy, Part I: The public health implications of variations in lactase persistence,* Journal of the National Medical Association, 1999, March; 91(3): 151-7.

Bishop, R.; *Science Behind Reported Benefits of Organic Milk,* Wisconsin Center for Dairy Research, June, 2007

Biswas, Akhil Bandhu; Chakraborty, Indranil; Das, Dillip Kumar; Biswas, Srabani; Nandy, Saswati; Mitra, Jayasri; *Iodine Deficiency Disorders among School Children of Malda, West Bengal, India.* Journal of Health, Population, and Nutrition, 2002, June; 20(2): 180-83

Bohmer, H.; Muller, H.; Resch, K.L.; *Calcium supplementation with calcium-rich mineral waters: a systematic review and meta-analysis of its bioavailability,* Osteoporosis International, 2000; 11(11): 938-43

Campbell, T. Colin; Campbell, T. M. II; *The China Study: The Most Comprehensive Study of Nutrition Ever Conducted and the Startling Implications for Diet, Weight Loss and Long Term Health*, Benbella Books, 2004

Cohen, R.; *Milk, The Deadly Poison,* Argus Publishing, Inc., 1998

docstoc; *Monsanto's History of Corruption, Manipulation, and Deception,* .docstoc, "Documents for Small Business & Professionals, www.docstoc.com/docs/29765410, 2010

DuPuis, M.; *Nature's Perfect Food, How Milk Became America's Drink,* New York University Press, 2002

Eaton, R.; *The Milk Imperative, A ticking bomb inside your body,* Published by DeliveredOnline.com, 2006

Eaton, S.B.; Konner, M.; *Paleolthic nutrition: A consideration of its nature and current implications,* The New England Journal of Medicine, 312(5): 283-89, www.ncbi.nlm.nih.gov/pubmed/2981409.

Eaton, S.B., Nelson, D.A.; *Calcium in evolutionary perspective,* The American Journal of Clinical Nutrition, 54(1 Suppl): 281S-287S, July, 1991.

Eaton, S.B.; Shostak, M.; Konner, M.; *The Paleolithic Prescription,* Harper & Row, 1988

Eaton, S.B., Eaton, S.B. III; Konner, M.J.; *Paleolithic nutrition revisited: A twelve-year retrospective on its nature and implications,* European Journal of Clinical Nutrition, 1997, 51, 207-216.

Epstein, S.S.; *What's In Your Milk?,* Trafford Publishing, 2006

Fenton, T.R.; Lyon, A.W.; Elasziw, M.; Tough, S.C.; Hanley, D.A.; *Meta-analysis of the effect of the acid-ash hypothesis of osteoporosis on calcium balance.* Journal of Bone and Mineral Research, 2009, November; 24(11): 1835-40.

Fogarty, P.; O'Beirne, B.; Casery, C.; *Epidemiology of the most frequent diseases in the European a-symptomatic post-menopausal women: Is there any difference between Ireland and the rest of Europe?*, Maturitas, 2005, November 15; Vol. 52, Supplement 1, Pages 3-6.

Food, Inc. Movie, *About the Film: How much do we really know about the food we buy at our local supermarkets and serve to our families?*, www.foodincmovie.com/about-the-film.php 2010

Godbole, N.N.; *Milk, The Most Perfect Food*, Biotech Books, 2007

Gratzer, Walter; *Terrors of the Table, The Curious History of Nutrition*, Oxford University Press, 2005.

Groff, J.L.; Gropper, S.S.; *Advanced Nutrition and Human Metabolism, Third Edition*, Wadsworth, 2000

Gropper, Sareen S.; Smith, J.L.; Groff, J.L.; *Advanced Nutrition and Human Metabolism, Fourth Edition*, Thomson/Wadsworth, 2005.

Grunwald, Michael; *Monsanto Held Liable for PCB Dumping*, Washington Post, February 23, 2002

Guthrie, H.A.; Picciano, M.F.; *Human Nutrition*, Mosby, 1998

Harris, Marvin; *Good To Eat, Riddles of Food And Culture*, Waveland Press, Inc, 1998

Holloway, Robert; *The Ancient Roots of Milk Consumption and its Genetic Dependence*, Nevada Technical Associates, Inc, 2009 www.ntanet.net/milk-consumption

International Farm Comparison Network (IFCN), *World Dairy Map 2009*, Results of the IFCN Dairy Report 2008. www.ifcndairy.org

IOF, International Osteoporosis Foundation ; *Policy and advocacy: Asia*, www.iofbonehealth.org/policy-advocacy/asia.htmn, May 15, 2010

IOF, International Osteoporosis Foundation; *Facts and statistics about osteoporosis and its impact*, www.iofbonehealth.org/facts-and-statistics.html May 15, 2010

IOM, Institute of Medicine, *Dietary Reference Intakes, The Essential Guide to Nutrient Requirements*, The National Academies Press, 2006

IOM, Institute of Medicine, *The Development of DRIs, 1994 – 2004, Lessons Learned and New Challenges, Workshop Summary*, The National Academies Press, 2008

Kikuch, Y.; Takebayashi, T.; Sasaki, S.; *Iodine concentration in current Japanese foods and beverages*, Nippon Eiseigaku Zasshi, 2008 July; 63(4): 724-34

Keon, J.; *Whole Health: The Guide to Wellness of Mind and Body, Diet Prevents Osteoporosis,* Parissound Publishing, 1997. Quoted by Jock Doubleday, Natural Woman, Natural Man, Inc. www.spontaneouscreation.org/SC/NWNM2006/DietPreventsOsteoporos is.htm

Kesse, E.; Bertrais, S.; Astorn, P.; Jaouen, A.; Arnault, N.; Galan, P.; Hercberg, S.; *Dairy products, calcium and phosphorus intake, and the risk of prostate cancer: results of the French prospective SU.VI.MAX (Supplementationen Vitamines et Mineraux Antioxydants) study,* British Journal of Nutrition, 2006, March: 95(3): 536-45.

Limpaphayom, K.K.; Taechakraichana, N.; Jaisamrarn, U.; Bunyavejchevin, S.; Chaikittisilpa, S.; Poshyachinda, M.; Taechamachai, C.; Havanond, P.; Onthuam,Y.; Lumbiganon, P.; Kamolratanakul, P.; *Prevalence of osteopenia and osteoporosis in Thai women,* Menopause, January, 2001, Vol. 8, Issue !: pp 65-69

Linger, Will; *U.S. and Europe Agree to Disagree on Safety of Dairy Hormone,* Press Release, June 30, 1999, by the Consumers Union, publisher of *Consumer Reports.*

McDougall, John A.; *The McDougall Plan,* New Win Publishing, Inc., 1983

MedHelp; *Lactose Intolerance,* www.medhelp.org/gov/www32.htm

Millward, D.J.; *Vernon Young and the development of current knowledge in protein and amino acid nutrition,* British Journal of Nutrition (In the press, 2004).

Montgomery, M.R.; *A Cow's Life,* Walker & Company, 2004

Morton, R.F.; Hebel, J.R.; McCarter, R.J.; *A Study Guide to Epidemiology and Biostatistis,* An Aspen Publication, 1996

National Family Health Survey (NFHS-3), India, 2005-06, compiled by Arnold, Fred; Parasuraman, Sulabha; Arokiasamy, P.; Kothari, Monica; Nutrition in India, International Institute for Population Sciences, Maryland, USA: ICF Macro

NOF (National Osteoporosis Foundation), *Fast Facts on Osteopororsis,* www.nof.org/osteoporosis/diseasefacts.htm May 6, 2010

Now Public, *Labeling rBHT milk,* www.nowpublic.com/health/labeling-rbht-milk May 23, 2010

OEN (OpEDNews), *Monsanto and Hillary Clinton's redemptive first act as Secretary of State,* www.opednews.com/articles/Monsanto-and-Hillary-Clint-by-Linn-Cohen-Cole-0902 May 23, 2010.

163

Organic Consumers Association, *98 Organizations Oppose Obama's Monsanto Man, Islam Siddiqui, for US Agricultural Trade Representative,* letter compiled by Dr. Marcia Ishii-Eiteman, Senior Scientist, Pesticides Action Network, and Katherine Ozer, Executive Director, National Family Farm Coalition, February 22, 2010.

Ornish, Dean; *Eat More, Weigh Less*, Harper Collins, 1994

Ornish, Dean; *Dr. Dean Ornish's Program for Reversing Heart Disease,* Ballantine Books, 1990

Oski, Frank, *M.D.; Don't Drink Your Milk*, Wyden Books, 1977

Pagano, M.; Gauvreau, K.; *Principles of Biostatistics,* Wadsworth, Inc., 1993

Pediatrics, *Policy Statement: Breastfeeding and the Use of Human Milk*, vol. 115, No. 2, February 2005, pp 496-506
www.aapolicy.aapublications.org

PCRM (Physicians Committee for Responsible Medicine); *PCRM Calls on the FTC to Investigate Misleading Health Claims in Milk ads,* PCRM News, 2010 www.pcrm.org/news/FTC_complaint.html

Philpott, Tom; *Conventional milk contains toxics, says the USDA,* The Organic Center (GRIST) www.grist.org/article/got-chemical-and-pesticide-residues-in-your-milk

PPJ Gazette, *American Farmers Cope With Roundup – Resistant Weeds (GM crops and superweeds)*, an article written by Willian Neuman and Andrew Pollack, May 6, 2010
www.ppjg.wordpress.com/2010/05/06/american-farmers-cope-with-roundup-resistant-weeds

Plant, Jane; *Your Life In Your Hands, Understanding, Preventing and Overcoming Breast Cancer,* Virgin Publishing Ltd, 2003.

Plant, J.; Tidey, G.; *Understanding, Preventing and Overcoming Osteoporosis*, Virgin Books, 2003

Ralson, S.H.; Uitterlinden, A.G.; *Genetics of Osteoprorosis,* Endocrine Review, April 29, 2010.

Smith, K.L.; *A Look at Physiological and Regulatory SCC Standards in Milk,* NMC Newsletter, "Udder Topics", December, 1997. Excerpted from a paper presented by K. Larry Smith, Ohio State University, at the International Dairy Federation (IDF) meeting in Vienna, Austria, September, 1995

Ramji, S.; *Iodine deficiency disorders-epidmiology, clinical profile and diagnosis.* In: Sachdev H.P.S.; Choudhury, P.; editors, Nutrition in children-developing countries conscern. New Delhi: Department of Paediatrics, Moulana Azad Medical College, 1995:245-54.

Raw Food Health, website: www.raw-food-health.net/NumberOfVegetarians.html 2010

Reinwald, S.; Weaver, C.M.; Kester, J.J.; *The health benefits of calcium citrate malate: a review of the supporting science,* Advanced Food Nurition Research, 2008; 54: 219-346

Remer, T.; Manz, F.; *Potential renal acid load of foods and its influence on urine pH,* Journal of the American Dietetic Association, 1995; 95: 791-97.

Rimas, A.; Fraser, E.D.G.; *Beef, The Untold Story of How Milk, Meat, and Muscle Shaped the World,* William Morrow, 2008

Robbins, John; *Diet For A New America,* Publishers Group West, 1987

Robbins, John; *The Food Revolution, How Your Diet Can Help Save Your Life And The World,* Cornell Press, 2001

Robbins, John; *The Truth About Calcium and Osteoporosis,* www.foodmatters.tv/_webapp_272927/The_Truth_About_Calcium_and_Osteoporosis, 2010

Rohmann, S.; Platz, E.A.; Kavanaugh, C.J.; Thuita, L.; Hoffman, S.C.; Helzisouer, K.J.; *Meat and dairy consumption and subsequent risk of prostate cancer in a US cohort study,* Cancer Causes & Control, 2007, February; 18(1): 41-50.

Scrimshaw, N.S.; *Human protein requirements: A brief update,* United Nations University Press, May 18, 2010 www.unu.edu/unupress/food/8F173e/8F173E02.htm

Scrimshaw, N.S.; Hussein, M.A.; Murray, E.; Rand, W.M.; Young, V.R.; *Protein requirements of man. Variations in obligatory urinary fecal losses in men,* Journal of Nutrition, 1972; 102; 1595-1604.

Scrimshaw, N.S.; Perera, W.D.; Young, V.R.; *Protein Requirements of Man: Obligatory Urinary and Fecal Nitrogen Losses in Elderly Women,* Journal of Nutrition, 106: 665-70, 1976

Segall, J.J.; *Dietary lactose as a possible risk factor for ischaemic heart disease: review of epidemiology,* International Journal of Cardiology, 1994, October; 46(3)

165

Shrier, I.; Szilagy, A.; Correa, J.A.; *Impact of lactose containing foods and the genetics of lactase on diseases: an analytical review of population data,* Nutrition and Cancer, 2008; 60(3): 292-309.

Spin Profiles, *Michael Taylor,* May 23, 2010
www.spinprofiles.org/indes.php/Michael_Taylor,

Stahler, Charles; *How many adults are vegetarian? The Vegetarian Resource Group asked in a 2006 national poll,* Vegetarian Journal, July-August, 2006. The poll was conducted by Harris Interactive.

Trevathan, W.R.; Smith, E.O.; McKenna, J.J.; *Evolutionary Medicine,* Oxford University Press, 1999

Tucker, K.L.; Hannan, M.T.; Kiel, D.P.; *The acid-base hypothesis: diet and bone in the Framingham Osteoporosis Study,* European Journal of Nutrition, 40: 231-237, 2001

United States Department of Agriculture (USDA),*National Nutrient Data base for Standard Reference, Release 22*, Nutrient Data Laboratory, Agricultural Research Service, http://www.nal.usda.gov/finic/foodcomp

Voegtlin, W.L.; *The stone age diet: Based on in-depth studies of human ecology and the diet of man,* Vantage Press, 1975

West, Keith P. Jr; *Extent of Vitamin A Deficiency among Preschool Children and Women of Reproductive Age*, The Journal of Nutrition, 132:2857S, September, 2002

WHO, *Population nutrient intake goals for preventing diet-related chronic diseases, 5.7.3: Diet, physical activity and osteoporosis,* www.who.int/nutrition/topics/5_population_nutrient/en/index25.html

Wikipedia, *Fast Food Nation (film)*, www.en.wikipedia.org/wiki/Fast-Food-Nation-(film), 2010

World Health Organization (WHO), *Elimination of iodine deficiency disorders in South East Asia*, Geneva, 1997:1-8. (SEA/NUT/138)

Young, Carl; *VA adds three more diseases to Agent Orange 'presumptive'list,* Times-Standard, November 18, 2009

Ziegler, E.E.; Filer, L.J. Jr.; editors; *Present Knowledge in Nutrition, Seventh Edition,* International Life Sciences Institiution, 1996, the article cited in this book is *Nutritional Advances in Osteoprorosis and Oteomalacia,* contributed by MaryFran Sowers.

WHO, World Health Organization, *Population nutrient intake goals for preventing diet-related chronic diseases,* May 15, 2010
www.who.int/nutrition/topics/5_population_nutrient/en/index25.html

Wikipedia, *Adelle Davis,* www.en.wikipedia.org/wiki/Adelle_Davis

Wikipedia, *Lactose intolerance, History of genetic prevalence,* www.en.wikipedia.org/wiki/Lactose_intolerance

Summary Statement for Chapter Three, the 'Bad'

Scientific research and studies that question the 'goodness' of milk are also plentiful, and also credible. Comparing the studies on the 'pro' side with those on the 'con' side makes clear that there is a great deal of controversy, complicated by our lack of knowledge in many areas. The influence of the existing paragdigm that venerates milk as 'nature's most perfect food may also be a key factor.

When studying the various research in favor of milk, I cannot help but ponder about how strong the influenc of this paradigm, or conventional wisdom, really is. I suspect that it is much stronger than one might imagine, and that the same research might end up very differently if carried out free of its influence.

This, then, promts me to give greater relative credibility to research that dares to challenge the prevailing paradigm and the proverbial goodness of milk.

One suggestion is that several earlier studies that indicate an association with milk consumption and disease conditions in humans may actually have identified the association with the A1 beta-casein variant (and BVM-7) in milk.

CHAPTER FOUR

'THE UGLY'

It is now suspected that the BCM7 peptide present in A1 milk causes an auto-immune reaction prompting T-cells to attack the insulin-producing beta cells in the pancreas, strongly promoting a diabetic condition. This same molecule may also act to oxidize LDL cholesterol and thus contribute to the formation of arterial plaque and heart disease. It may, in addition, pass through the blood-brain-barrier and effect neurological processes leading to schizophrenia, autism, sudden-death syndrome, and other neurological disorders.

Devil in the milk

The BCM-7 hypothesis may never have been presented to the public arena had it not been for the effort and writings of one individual, Dr. Keith Woodford. A Professor of Farm Management and Agribusiness at the Lincoln University in New Zealand, Dr. Woodford has been a relentless searcher for the truth in this newly emerging field of study and inquiry. He published *Devil In The Milk; Illness, Health, and the Politics of A1 and A2 Milk* in 2007, with a follow-up North American edition in 2009. His book is an in-depth review and analysis of the pertinent scientific research, the creation of A2 Corporation and its role, the mischievous counter-effort by the New Zealand dairy industry, and the head-in-the-sand attitude of the New Zealand and EU governments.

I urge my readers to read *Devil In The Milk* ... it is fascinating and enlightening reading. At various points I have expanded on Dr. Woodford's work, and have included some additional information. But I rely heavily on what he has written in his compelling expose'. I have also decided not to review or reference *all* of the numerous research studies and articles which he has already presented in his book ... but will only introduce those that are most directly related. I have, however, referenced additional studies that have been published since his 2007 writing.

It is probably appropriate that Dr. Woodford refers to the BCM-7 molecule as a *devil*, and as he adds, it is indeed a *tricky little devil*.

1. The BCM-7 Hypothesis: A Chronology

It was in the year 1997, and I was studying nutrition at the University of Hawaii … I had just read a research study by Karjalainan et el (1992) in the New England Medical Journal that suggested that a peptide in cow's milk can attach to the surface protein of the human pancreas beta-cell, thus provoking an autoimmune response resulting in the destruction of the beta-cell. The pancreas beta cell is the source of insulin which controls the glucose sugar uptake by the body's cells … damage to the beta cells can therefore lead to diabetes. I mentioned this article to one of my professors a few days later, and to my dismay I was strongly admonished for not being more critical of my selected reading.

It was clear than my professor knew nothing of this new area of research at the time … and there was nothing that I could find in my textbooks on the subject either. In fact, this was then only a maverick concept, and only a small number of scientists worldwide were beginning to put together the many intricate pieces of the puzzle.

The beginning of the BCM-7 story

Yes, one of the most fascinating characteristics of science is that the individual pieces of a bigger picture, or puzzle, are slowly and painstakingly worked out, bit by bit, piece by piece, no one really understanding how they will finally come together until after the fact. And that is how it is with the BCM-7 story.

It has been suspected for a very long time that something in cow's milk was the cause of ill health in humans. One condition was identified as *cow's milk allergy*, and concern for this illness prompted the movement to promote breast-feeding, beginning in the early 1970s. Even during that decade it was recognized that the problem lay with the protein in milk, possibly with the casein portion.

A1 and A2 milk

Knowledge of the differences between breeds of dairy cattle and the characteristics of their milk go back to the time that humans first domesticated the lineage of the cow, beginning with the ancient *auroch*, or *Bos primigenius,* the giant primordial ox. Extensive selective breeding, cross-breeding, and the occurrence of mutations over the millennia have greatly modified and expanded that single beginning. There are now about 920 dairy cattle breeds worldwide, including many exotic breeds surviving in remote areas. However, most modern-day dairy cattle belong to the humpless sub-species *Bos taurus,* which is further divided into *Bos taurus indicus*, adapted to hot climates, and *Bos taurus taurus*, adapted to cooler climates. Six breeds predominate in the United States and most of the Western countries, which are the Ayrshire, the Brown Swiss, the Guernsey, Jersey, Milking Shorthorn, and the Holstein-Friesian. The Aryshire, originally from Scotland, is known for their hardiness; the small Jersey and Guernsey for the high cream *and* high protein content of their milk; and the familiar black and white Holstein-Friesian is known for its un-matched high production. The Holstein-Friesian , originally from Germany, is the predominant breed in the U.S. and Europe. The milk produced by each of these many different breeds varies considerably in content, and the content can also be influenced by feed and local environmental factors.

As reviewed in Chapter One, the major protein in cow's milk is *casein*, which comprises 76 to 86% of the total milk protein, and is divided into alpha-casein, beta casein, and gamma casein, with alpha casein being the major portion (60% of the total casein). Alpha casein is further separated into 'alpha-s-casein' and 'k-casein'. The remaining 14 to 24% of the protein portion in milk is a variety of proteins collectively called 'whey proteins', of which *lactoglobulin* is the most common (7-12% of the total whey proteins). For our discussion of the BCM-7 molecule, however, the genetic differences in the casein protein portion of the cow's milk is where we draw attention to.

Of the casein protein portion, 27% is 'beta casein', with as many as 15 different variations found among the milks produced by the world's dairy cattle population, with the variations dependent on the separate cattle species and breeds. All beta casein from all cow breeds, however, is comprised of a folded chain of 209 individual amino acids. Genetically, and historically, the original beta casein amino acid sequence in cow's milk contained a 'proline' at position number 67. But the first sequence discovered via modern scientific investigation found a 'histidine' at that position, and thus this variation was named A1. We now know that the original variation contained a 'proline' amino acid at position 67, but this version has never-the-less been dubbed the A2 variant. The switch to a histidine at position 67 is thought to be due to a mutation which presumably occurred among one single breed or species a few thousand years ago …which we now know is the Friesian/Holstein breed originating from Europe.

In my research of early scientific knowledge about the genetic variations in cow's milk, and in particular about variations in the casein protein, I found that scientific investigation into the variations goes back to at least 1961, with a study by R. Aschaffenburg entitled *Inherited casein variants in cow's milk.* In 1963 the same researcher published *Inherited casein variants in cow's milk. II. Breed differences in the occurrence of β-casein variants.* During the following year, 1964, a study by Thompson et al entitiled *Genetic polymorphism in caseins of cow's milk. II. Confirmation of the genetic control of beta-casein variations* confirmed Aschaffenburg's work. Five variations of the beta-casein in cow's milk were isolated, and were initially categorized as A, B, C, D, E, and F, reflecting the order in which they were identified.

An excellent 19-page review of the discoveries of the many variations of milk proteins in all the sub-species of *Bos genus* is presented by Formaggioni et al in their 1999 paper entitled *Milk Protein Polymorphism: Detection and Diffusion of the Genetic Variants in Bos Genus.* In their review they credit Aschaffenburg with identifying and naming the 'A' variety of β-casein with his 1961 and 1963 studies, and then credits Peterson et al and Kiddy et al with first identifying a change of the amino acid at position 67 of the β-casein, from Proline to Histidine, and a change from histidine to glycine at position 106. The A type β-casein was thus separated into A1 (with the histidine at position 67), A2 (with proline at position 67), and A3 (with glycine at position 106 instead of histidine). Their work was published in 1966.

In Table 3 of Formaggioni et al's paper, it shows that the change of position 67 from a proline to a histidine also occurred in other varieties of β-casein, and identifies the research that led to each of the findings. Although Aschaffenburg was not aware of the differences in 'A' β-casein that would lead to the separation into A1, A2, and A3, he *had* discovered that β-casein 'B' and 'C' also had the histidine at position 67, which he discovered at the same time that he isolated β-casein 'A'. However, with 'B' β-casein there was also a switch from serine to arginine at position 122. With 'C' β-casein there was also a switch from glucine to lysine at position 37, and a switch from serine P to serine at position 35.

Then, some 17 years later, two more β-casein variants were added ... 'G' and 'H', and it was further discovered that the 'H' variant had the histidine instead of proline at position 67 as well ... discovered by Han et al in 1983 and confirmed by Chung et al in 1995, and again by Han et al in 1996. Visser et al found that the 'F' β-casein also had the same change (1991 and 1995); and Chin & Ng-Kwai-Hang found that variant 'G' again had the histidine at position 67 (1997) … their work was confirmed by Dong & Ng-Kwai-Hang in 1998.

By 1999 it was therefore known that the β-casein variants that included a histidine at position 67 included A1, B, C, F, G, and H.

However, it was recognized that the most significant occurrence of the histidine instead of a proline at position 67 lay with the A1 β-casein, which accounted for the greater part of modern milk production. The case of 'B' β-casein may be an interesting secondary concern … the 'B' β-casein is relatively common in some parts of Europe.

Other researchers followed suit confirming the early work with A1, A2, and A3 variants by Aschaffenburg, Peterson & Kopfler, and Kiddy. By 1984 many scientists and researchers were well versed with the concept of the A1, A2, and A3 variations of beta casein protein in milk, and understood that these variations were dependent on genetics. An example is the 1984 study by Ng-Kwai-Hang et al, entitled *Association of genetic variants of casein and milk serum proteins with milk, fat, and protein production by dairy cattle.* Ng-Kwai-Hang and his research team are noted for their additional work in this field. For example, one of their contributions is Chapter 16 of the well-known textbook *Advanced Dairy Chemistry* (2002). The chapter was entitled *Genetic polymorphism of milk protein,* which provides an authoritative 78-page overview of the genetic variants in milk proteins and the history of their discovery.

One question that has popped is "Why did the mutation that produced the histidine in place of a proline at position 67 survive … was it somehow beneficial for the animal?" A good question. We do not know if, or how this mutation would benefit the animal, but another explanation makes some sense. The opioid peptide (BCM-7) generated by the variant with the histidine at position 67, when fed to the cow's young, and perhaps passed on from generation to generation, would likely render the animals more passive and easier to handle. Thus the mutation was beneficial to the human agriculturist, rather than the animal, in assisting in domestication and animal husbandry.

The casein peptides

With digestion of beta casein in the human stomach and small intestine, the protein chain is first broken down into fragments, or 'peptides'. With the 209 amino acid sequence, the break-down into separate fragments can potentially create a large number of individual peptides. Many of these peptides are 'biologically active', which means that they can have a biological effect on physiological processes within the human body. A number of these peptides are known to play beneficial and protective roles, others can be outright *devilish*. Beneficial effects include improved digestion, protection from cardiovascular disease, enhanced immune defense, and benefits to nervous system processes.

The different genetic variants of the casein protein also affect how the 209 amino acid chain fragments, or breaks up. Several digestive enzymes act to facilitate the separation, such as 'pepsin', 'leucine amino peptidase' and 'pancreatic elastase'. The amino acid proline tends to stabilize the chain at that point and keeps it intact, while the amino acid histidine allows the chain to fold, and easily break at its location. Several prolines close together tend to make that section exceptionally stable and resistant to further fragmentation. One important example is the proline or histidine at position number 67. With the proline at position 67 the chain will tend to separate in that area of the chain to form three specific peptides which are noted for their beneficial effect: (a) the ten amino acid peptide from position 57 through 66 which is known to inhibit one enzyme that is linked to aggravating neurological disorders, (b) the six amino acid peptide containing positions 59 through 64, which is known to lower blood pressure, and (c), the five amino acid peptide containing positions 59 through 63, which demonstrates a role in enhancing the body's immune response. However, with a switch from the proline to a histidine at position 67 these three peptides are prevented from separating … instead the usual peptides separated are a seven-amino acid fragment containing positions 60 through 66, and a truncated form of this same peptide containing positions 60 through 64. The amino acid sequence in the seven long chain is Tyrosine-Proline-Phenylalanine-Proline-Glycine-Proline-Isoleucine. It is also important to note that the last 4 amino acids in this sequence, numbers 60-66, are Proline-Glysine-Proline-Isoleucine.

During the 89s and 90s a number of studies investigated which casein peptide could possibly be the connection to 'cow;s milk allergy'. Several peptides were targeted as the potential *devil*. One peptide was the 17 amino-acid chain 'bovine serum albumin peptide (ABBOS), first identified by Karjalainen et al in 1993. This peptide is still being much studied.

The β- casomorphins, and BCM-7

"Caso" meaning "like" and "morphin", short for "morphine". In 1979 Henschen et al (H. Teschemacher was the team leader), published a paper entitled *Novel opioid peptides derived from casein (beta-casomorphins)*.

II. Structure of active components from bovine peptone. This was the first finding that the casein peptide fragments were 'casein-casomorphins' ... in other words, were opioid-active peptide fragments. These peptides, thus, had opiate properties similar to that of the narcotics, opium and morphine. One of the casomorphins identified in the Teschemacher study was the 'beta-casomorphin-7' peptide, the peptide fragment containing positions 60 through 66. "Beta-casomorphin-7" was eventually abbreviated to BCM-7 (although just when I couldn't determine) ... and yes, *this is the BCM-7 ... the devil in the milk !!* Teschemacher concluded in his study that these casomorphins were highly bioactive and may be associated with promoting disease conditions in humans.

The opiate-like beta-casomorphins contain anywhere from 4 to 11 amino acids in their chain, and all start with tyrosine followed by a proline, and have another tyrosine or a phenylalanine in the third or fourth position. This is known to be an important structural form which fits or matches the binding sites of opioid receptors in the human body. With this structure the peptide can attach to receptors in the body that then enable opiate-related activity. It is noted that the removal of the tyrosine completely inhibits bioactivity.

The BCM-7 casomorphin is exceptionally potent. For example, it takes ten times the amount of the drug 'naloxone', which is used to counter the effects of morphine overdose, to counteract an equivalent amount of BCM-7. A five amino acid truncated form of beta casomorphin-7, dubbed BCM-5, exhibits an even stronger opiate effect. The drug naloxone is often used in studies to test the presence of BCM-7 or BCM-5 and their opiate effect.

BCM-7 and A1, A2 milk

We can now begin to pull the knowledge of A1 and A2 milk together with what we know about the BCM-7 peptide. We know that the seven amino acid chain (the BCM-7 segment) is highly unlikely to separate intact if the amino acid at position 67 is a proline, as in the A2 genetic variant ... the original variant for *Bos taurus*. However, when this position is occupied by the amino acid histine, the chain folds at that point and the fragment 60 through 66 easily separates ... and position 67 is a histine in the A1, B, C, F, G, and H casein variants.

Kaminski et al (2007) lists six beta-casomorphins naturally occurring in bovine milk plus two in human milk. Yes, human milk also has beta-casomorphins ... BCM-7 and BCM-8. The main difference is that the

174

second proline position in bovine BCM-7 is a valine in human BCM-7, and the amino acid after the end isoleucine is a proline in human milk instead of a histidine. Thus human BCM-7 acts like an A2 peptide rather than an A1 peptide, and the opioid effect is greatly reduced. The six bovine beta-casomorphins listed are BCM-4, BCM-5, BCM-6, BCM-7, BCM-8, and BCM-11.

Milk production and BCM-7

The dairy cow carries the gene that determines its casein variant on the sixth chromosome. These variants can be divided into the A1, B, C, F, G, and H variants which have a histidine at position 67 and can therefore produce the BCM-7 peptide ... and the A2, A3, D, and E variants which have a proline at position 67 and therefore cannot produce the BCM-7 peptide. The proline at position 67 is the original variant ... the histidine at that position is theoretically due to a mutation that occurred with a specific breed in Europe several thousand years ago.

Dairy breeds vary greatly in respect to their casein variant, but for the 6 most common breeds in Western countries, the Holstein-Freisian is the most likely to produce milk with the BCM-7 molecule. The next most likely are the Ayrshire, Jersey, and Milking Shorthorn, which can all be ranked as equal. The next least likely is the Brown Swiss, and then the Guernsey is the least likely of all. There are also a number of breeds that are more specific to one locality, and these breeds are often of the A2, D, and E variant. Two interesting examples are the 'Normande' breed of France and the 'Icelandic Cow' or 'Norske' of Iceland. Both the French and Icelandic breeds are historically ancient, with little or no prior inter-breeding with dairy cattle from other countries. India is another example of a country that has a number of exotic dairy breeds; many of which also belong to the A2, D, and E variant group.

For the sake of convenience, and because the majority of the A1, B, C, F, G, and H casein variants being produced worldwide today is A1 and B, we can simply call this group 'A1/B', or even just 'A1'. Similarly, we can shorten the A2, A3, D, and E group to 'A2'.

The prevalence of breeds in the dairy stock of individual counties varies greatly, as does the total cow population. In this respect New Zealand stands out. With a total human population of 4.23 million in 2007, the total dairy cow population was almost the same ... a whopping 4.20 million ... one dairy cow for every member of the population. The national dairy herd in 2007 was made up of 47% Holstein-Friesian, 15%

Jersey, 2% Ayrshire, and the rest a mixture of Guernsey, Brown Swiss, and Meuse Rhine Issel.

The Holstein-Friesian is a magnificent milking animal. They are large, stylish animals with color patterns of black and white, and sometimes red and white. A mature cow weighs about 1,500 pounds and stands 58 inches tall at the shoulder. Average annual production per animal in 2009 was 23,151 pounds of milk, 842 pounds of butterfat, and 711 pounds of protein. Top producing Holstein-Friesians are milked three times a day and have been known to produce in excess of 72,000 pounds of milk in 365 days. In the United States, more than 19 million Holstein-Friesians are registered in the American Holstein Association's Herdbook, and account for more than 90% of the total dairy stock in the U.S.

As mentioned, the dairy cow carries the gene that determines its casein variant on the sixth chromosome. If we simplify the variants to A1 or A2, the trait for whether a cow will produce A1 or A2 beta casein is carried in the genes it inherits from its mother and father ... one gene is inherited from each parent for the trait of beta casein production, and thus each cow carries two genes determining what form of beta casein it produces. Cows can have only the A1 or only the A2 production trait, or they can have one of each.

The breed of the cow also plays an important role in this respect... the proportion of A1 to A2 beta casein in the cow's milk varies between the breeds of cows. For example, in the Holstein-Friesian, the most common trait distribution is:

- A quarter of the cows will carry traits for the production of A1 beta-casein, without the trait for A2, and will therefore produce only A1 milk.
- Half of the cows will carry a combination of traits for the production of both A1 and A2 beta-casein, and their milk will therefore be a 50 – 50 mix of A1 and A2.
- A quarter of the cows will carry traits for the production of A2 beta-casein, without the trait for A1, and will therefore produce only A2 milk.

This means, then, that 25% of milk from the Holstein-Friesian will be A1, 50% a 50 -50 mix of A1 and A2, and 25% only A2. However, unless care is taken to separate the pure A2 from the A1 and mixed A1/A2 milk, which is not normally done, the milks will be mixed in the holding tanks both at the farm and at the dairy. This then means that just about 100% of the mixed milk produced by the Holstein-Friesian will contain at least some A1 beta casein and will have the potential to produce the BCM-7 peptide. The exception will possibly be milk that is specifically kept separate from the bulk of the milk coming from the farms … milk that is from Gurnseys and Jerseys, for example, which is high in cream content and/or protein content, or milk that is identified as A2 instead of A1 or a mixture. However, there is no effort in the U.S. or Europe at the present time to identify and/or to separate the two variants of milk. This is only being done in New Zealand and Australia, and even in those countries only on a small scale.

Woodford reports that in 2007 A2 milk was made available in 'Hy-Vee' supermarkets in seven mid-western states in the U.S. But in December, 2008 the A2 Milk Company announced that they were withdrawing A2 products from sale pending a new marketing strategy. There is currently no A2 milk commercially available in the United States. One issue was that the A2 milk was "certified to contain at least 2 grams of A2 type beta-casein per serving". This implies that *not all the beta-casein was variant A2*, and so our BCM-7 devil could still be lurking in that glass of so-called A2 milk purchased at the Hy-Vee supermarket.

With 90% of the dairy cattle in the US being Holstein-Friesian, combined with the universal practice of mixing milks in holding tanks, almost all the milk currently sold commercially in the United States contains some A1, with the likelihood of it containing at least 50% A1.

An agreement between A2 Corporation and Purmil of Korea to market A2 milk in that country under the label 'Lotte' was terminated in December, 2009.

How does BCM-7 from A1 beta-casein enter the body ??

The BCM-7 peptide fragment derived from type A1 beta-casein is broken off from the 209 amino acid chain during normal digestion in the human stomach and small intestine. It is a relatively large molecule, however, and does not normally pass through the membranes of the small intestine wall. This had been a highly debated factor giving support to the argument that the BCM-7 molecule cannot and does not present a health issue … simply because it does not enter the blood stream with normal digestion. This also may help to explain why the effects of the BCM-7 molecule have remained hidden from scientific investigation for so long.

However, this is still controversial … there are a few studies that suggest that the BCM-7 molecule *can* pass through the small intestine lining under even normal digestion conditions. For example, Iwan et al

(2008), in their study entitled *Transport of micro-opioid receptor agonists and antagonist peptided across Caco-2 monolayer,* investigated whether beta-casomorphins could pass through one specific area of the small intestine membrane, named Caco-2. They found that they could, indeed, pass through. The BCM-7 beta-casomorphin was one of the peptides tested.

Sienkiewicz-Szlapka et al confirmed the results of the Iwan et al study in their very recent publication entitled *Transport of bovine milk-derived opioid peptides across a Caco-2 monolayer* (April, 2009), published in the International Dairy Journal.

It is also known that the enzyme 'dipeptidyl peptidase 4' (DPP4), located on the intestine mesenteric tissue, can act to degrade the BCM-7 molecule and break it down into smaller segments, such as the even stronger opioid BCM-5, which can pass through the intestinal lining more easily.

In addition, we know that the BCM-7 molecule can easily enter the blood stream if any of a variety of special conditions exist. The most important of these special conditions is common with infants ... the digestive system of the newborn human baby is not fully developed and remains permeable to the transport of large molecules across the small intestine wall for at least the first six months, and often into early childhood. This means that the BCM-7 molecule readily transfers into the blood stream of babies.

In addition, persons may have what is termed a 'leaky gut' for a number of reasons and conditions, and this will also allow the BCM-7 molecule to enter the blood stream. These conditions include Coeliac disease, ulcerative colitis, Crohn's disease, and stomach ulcers. It is interesting to note that a common treatment of stomach ulcers has been to drink milk ... one example is the 'Sippy' high milk diet, which has also been related to an increased incidence of deaths due to heart disease. It is also worthy of mention that it has been found that individuals suffering from various neurological disorders, such as autism and schizophrenia, often have unusually permeable digestive systems, although this claim has been contested.

The diabetes and milk connection

The possible association of the BCM-7 molecule with diabetes refers to 'insulin-dependent diabetes mellitus', or IDDM. This form of diabetes is more commonly called Type 1 diabetes, or juvenile-onset diabetes.

Other forms of diabetes include Type 2 diabestes, or 'late-onset diabetes', and 'gestational diabetes' (GDM), which is a form of carbohydrate intolerance. Both of these two other forms can be treated through dietary changes and health care.

Type 1 diabetes accounts for 10-15% of all people with the disease. It can appear at any age, although most commonly with infants, children, and juveniles. People with Type 1 diabetes must inject themselves with insulin several times a day and must follow a careful diet and exercise plan.

An autoimmune response refers to the action by the body's immune system to isolate and attack invading substances. More specifically, antibodies, or 'T-cells', are produced by the body's immune system to attack 'antigens', or foreign viruses, bacteria, or other harmful compounds. The presence of an antigen stimulates the immune system to produce these antibodies, which then attack the antigens, inactivating them, and helping to remove them from the body. While antigens can be from pathogenic (diseases-causing) infections and viruses, they can also be organic molecules from internal or environmental sources. Once the immune system has created an antibody for an antigen whose attack it has survived, it continues to produce antibodies to protect from further attacks by that same antigen.

Diabetes is a disorder of metabolism which interferes with the way the body uses digested food for growth and energy. A major part of the food we eat is broken down to synthesize glucose, the form of sugar in the blood. Glucose is the main sources of fuel for the body. Once in the blood stream, glucose is distributed to the various cells for uptake. A hormone produced by the pancreas (insulin) is required to be present to initiate and control the uptake of glucose by the individual cells. The pancreas is a large gland positioned behind the stomach, and it is the beta-cells in the pancreas that produce the needed insulin. After food digestion the right amount of insulin to move glucose from the blood into the cells is secreted. In people with insulin-dependent diabetes mellitus, however, the beta-cells malfunction, or don't function at all, and either too little or no insulin is generated. Uptake of glucose into the cells is thus diminished, and glucose levels in the blood rise. As a consequence glucose spills into the urine and is excreted from the body. In this situation the body loses its main source of fuel and energy ... even though the blood contains large amounts of glucose ... and a disease condition results. IDDM becomes clinically symptomatic when approximately 80 –

85% of the pancreatic beta-cells are destroyed, requiring insulin injection as an intervention measure.

Classical symptoms of IDDM, or Type 1 diabetes include increased hunger and frequent urination. Prolonged high glucose levels causes 'glucose absorption' and effects such as a change in vision due to excess glucose altering the shape of the eye lenses. A number of skin rashes can occur with diabetes, collectively known as 'diabetic dermadr'. A form of 'ketoacidosis' is also common, characterized by the smell of acetone. Rapid, deep breathing, nausea, vomiting, and an altered state of consciousness can be additional symptoms. Diabetics often experience wound-healing problems, and swelling of the extremities. Amputation of arms or legs can be an extreme consequence, and even death.

The concept that insulin-dependent diabetes mellitus could be caused by the destruction of pancreatic beta-cells by an autoimmune response is also not new. The 81-page PhD dissertation by Paula Klemetti (1999) gives an excellent review of the literature and studies up to that time, and tells us that W. Gepts in his study entitled *Pathologic anatomy of the pancreas in juvenile diabetes mellitus*, was the first to identify the role of autoimmune mechanisms in the destruction of the pancreatic beta-cells, leading to IDDM. That was in 1965. During the 70s, 80s, and 90s a large number of studies were conducted which addressed the autoimmune link with diabetes.

The consensus in the scientific community now concludes that Type 1 diabetes is characterized by the destruction of the insulin-producing beta cells in the pancreas by the body's own immune system. The immune system reaction which causes the beta cells to be attacked is known to be potentially triggered by a number of possible factors, including genetic, disease, and environmental factors. The environmental factors, in turn, can include viruses, and diet. Suggested dietary factors, to take this one more step, have included wheat gluten and various milk proteins. Yes, milk proteins ... which potentially could be whey protein or casein protein.

One must therefore appreciate that IDDM is a multi-factoral disease condition, and although the immune response mechanism has been isolated as the central probable cause, the trigger to the initiation of this mechanism could be the result of any of a number of factors ... which include milk protein.

By sometime in the early 1980s two very separate pieces of our puzzle were therefore apparent, yet were so far removed and had emerged from such different fields of study that the connection was not realized. It was known that (1) there were differences in the make-up of the casein protein in milk and that strongly bioactive peptides could be generated, and (2) that the mechanism leading to insulin-dependent diabetes mellitus was probably the destruction of the pancreas beta-cells by an autoimmune attack. But putting the two concepts together had not been thought of.

How the auto-immune attack was triggered was a central question at the time. One clue presented itself during this period, however, and that was the fact that infants and young children with IDDM frequently and consistently had residues of milk protein antigens and the corresponding antibodies within their blood stream. The presence of specific milk protein antigens and their matching antibodies in infants with IDDM strongly suggested a causal link between the consumption of milk protein and the onset of IDDM in infants. These studies were used during those earlier years as support for the promotion of breastfeeding, and also to encourage manufacturers of commercial infant formulas to process the milk proteins to render them less reactive biologically. At the time the main concern was *cow's milk allergy*. It was thought that only infants with certain conditions which led to high risk were susceptible. Investigators did not, however, associate the allergy condition with any specific milk variety, although milk caseins were then suspected to be the source.

Along comes Robert Elliott

Robert Elliot and Martin, in their 1984 study *Dietary proteins: a trigger of insulin-dependent diabetes in the BB rat?* were the first to find evidence that the antigen prompting the autoimmune mechanism that Gepts had identified back in 1965 was a protein contained in cow's milk (at that time termed 'CM proteins').

Professor Bob Elliott was a diabetes researcher at Auckland University in New Zealand and was working mostly with animal models, particularly the BB rat, which is a rat breed known to be especially susceptible to the onset of diabetes. With his beginning studies Elliott knew that milk protein was strongly linked with promoting diabetes in the BB rat, but it was not clear which protein was the culprit, nor was Elliott aware of the different genetic variants in the milk proteins, particularly casein.

During the late 1980s and 90s a number of studies continued to investigate which milk protein could be the connection to human autoimmune reactions and disease risk, particularly IDDM. Several milk proteins were targeted as the potential antigen, and different mechanisms were hypothesized. One outstanding study was by Dahl-Jergensen et al (1991), which was also referenced in Chapter Three. Another example was a number of studies generated by the Childhood Diabetes in Finland Study. Two of these have also been listed in the additional reference section of the previous chapter (Virtanen et al, 1998, 2000).

One of the protein peptides investigated was the 17 amino-acid chain 'bovine serum albumin peptide (ABBOS), first identified by Karjalainen et al in 1993. Another was the 7-amino acid segment in β-casein at positions 60 through 66 ... the BCM-7 peptide.

Keith Woodford reports in his book, *Devil In The* Milk, that sometime in 1993 Professor Robert Elliott telephoned the New Zealand Dairy Research Institute (NZDRI), asking to speak to someone who knew about cows and milk-protein biochemistry. Dr. Jeremy Hill took the call. The question was: is there a significant chemical difference in the proteins of milk from different cows ?? Hill then clarified that, yes, there is indeed a difference, which can separate the milk into two broad categories: A1 milk and A2 milk. Elliott then compared the incidence of IDDM with his mice, feeding them A1 and A2 milk. In his preliminary study, all the mice fed A1 milk developed IDDM and died. None of the mice fed A2 milk became diabetic.

It is interesting to note that the A1 and A2 milk samples used by Elliott in his work with mice was supplied by the New Zealand Dairy Research Institute, with funding from the New Zealand Dairy Board. In addition, Jeremy Hill, from NZDRI, was a co-researcher in those early studies.

One of Elliot's population studies during that same period compared Samoan children living in New Zealand with children living in their native homeland. Children in Samoa at the time consumed almost no milk, but Samoan children living in New Zealand did ... a lot ... like other New Zealanders. He found a ten-fold difference in the incidence of diabetes between the two children groups.

But he also knew that the incidence of diabetes varies greatly between countries ... as much as by a factor of more than 300 ... and that the variation could not be explained by *total* milk consumption alone. Finland, for example, consumes the highest amount of cow's milk and has the highest incidence of diabetes. But the populations of nearby France and Iceland also consume high amounts of bovine milk, yet have much lower rates of diabetes. This is especially true with Iceland. He had also studied the Masai people of Kenya, who consumed very large quantities of cow's milk, yet had an almost non-existent incidence of type 1 diabetes.

With his new knowledge of the difference between A1 and A2 milk Robert Elliot was thus pointed in the direction of undertaking further epidemiological studies in human populations to specifically compare diabetes and other diseases with the consumption of these two different types of milk.

The Pozzilli study

In 1996 Cavallo et al (Pozzilli was their team leader) studied the beta-casein peptides, in particular the position 60-66 in the 209 amino-acid beta-casein chain. They made a remarkable discovery: the 4-amino-acid sequence at the end of the 7-amino acid fragment was the same as the number 415 – 419 residues of the pancreas beta-cell glucose transporter molecule, named GLUT-2. This amino acid sequence was Proline-Glysine-Proline-Isoleucine (as noted in a previous section). Cavallo and Pozzilli were thus the first to recognize that this particular peptide fragment possessed special characteristics that made it a candidate for a possible role in an autoimmune reaction, specifically a reaction involving the pancreas beta-cells. They suggested that the antibodies attacking the cow's milk casein fragment with the 60 – 66 amino-acid sequence would inadvertently also attack the GLUT-2 molecule in the beta-cell, thus rendering the beta-cell function inoperable.

Pozzillis' reputation as a scientist and a specialist in the field of diabetes is impeccable. The reference at the end of the chapter highlights some of his achievements. His work lended considerable credibility to the BCM-7 – GLUT-2 proposed mechanism. Additional support, as already mentioned, came from a long list of studies that were carried out in the 70s, 80s, and early 90s that observed the presence of beta-casein antigens and matching antibodies in infants with IDDM that had been fed cow's milk, or commercial formula based on cow's milk. The study by Karjalainem et al which I encountered during my undergraduate studies at UH was one such study.

Additional studies during this period

Besides peer review of published studies, scientists often share their findings and research data among peers and associates. News of Elliott's work apparently spread, and generated interest and other studies. One example is a study by I. Thorsdottir and O. Reykdal of Iceland in 1997 entitled *Food and the low incidence of IDDM in Iceland*. Their conclusion was as follows:

"The incidence of IDDM is lower in Iceland than among the genetically related nations of Scandinavia. Recent animal research in New Zealand has pinpointed a specific protein fraction in cow's milk, A1 β-casein, as one of the possible causes of an immunological destruction of the pancreatic β-cells resulting in IDDM. Milk protein allele frequencies in the Nordic cattle breeds varies, and preliminary results indicate that A1 β-casein is especially low in Icelandic milk."

Thorsdottir's completed a second study entitled *Different β-caseub fractions in Icelandic versus Scandinavian cow's milk may influence diabetogenicity of cow's milk in infancy and explain low incidence of insulin-dependent diabetes mellitus in Iceland.* Jeremy Hill was listed as one of the seven authors, and the study was published in the journal Pediatrics in 2000. The conclusion to this study was:

"The lower fraction of A1 and B β-casein in Icelandic cow's milk may explain why there is a lower incidence of IDDM in Iceland than in Scandinavia."

A third study, again with Jeremy hill, was published in 2002 and was entitled *Variations in consumption of cow milk proteins and lower incidence of Type 1 diabetes in Iceland vs the other 4 Nordic countries.* The conclusion was: "... A1 and B beta-casein may contribute to varying diabetolgenicity of cow's milk and explain the difference in incidence of Type 1 diabetes." (Birgisdottir et al, 2002)

Thorsdottir showed up once more as co-author of a study entitled *Lower consumption of cow milk protein A1 beta-casein at 2 years of age, rather than consumption among 11- to 14-year old adolescents, may explain the lower incidence of type 1 diabetes in Iceland than in Scandinavia,* and was published in the journal Annals of Nutrition and Metabolism, 2006 (Birgisdottir et al, 2006). The title of the study is also their conclusion. This conclusion makes sense, considering that infants exhibit a more permeable digestive system with allows the BCM-7 casomorphin peptide to enter the blood stream.

It should also be noted that Jeremy Hill was one of the total of four authors (once again). Hill was with Fonterra at the time of Thorsdittir's fourth study, and Fonterra was then engaged in all-out war with A2 Corporation and the entire A1/A2 (BCM-7) hypothesis.

I refer to these studies, and the authors, in a later section ... Thorsdottir later became one of the authors of the 2009 EFSA Report.

Professor Robert Elliott returns

In 1999 Elliott and his research team completed and published a study entitled *Type 1 (insulin-dependent) diabetes mellitus and cow milk: casein variant consumption*. The study built on previous work comparing IDDM in 0 to 14-year-old children from 10 countries, using national annual cow milk protein consumption data. Their finding was that although total protein consumption did not correlate with the incidence of diabetes, consumption of the beta-casein A1 variant definitely did. The 'correlation coefficient was $r = 0.726$. Even more pronounced was the relation between beta-casein 'A1+B' consumption and IDDM, with a correlation coefficient of $r = 0.928$. As I stated in the previous paragraphs, the 'B' variant of β-casein can also produce the seven amino acid β-casein peptide fragment from positions 60 through 66 (BCM-7). Milk containing the B variant of β-casein was relatively common in the populations he targeted. The calculated degree of correlation is nothing short of astonishing.

It was not until 2003, however, that Elliot and his co-worker, Laugesen, were able to complete a larger between-country correlation study and finally draw a higher level of attention to their research. They compared mortality (death rate) due to ischaemic heart disease (HCD) and the incidence of Type 1 insulin-dependent diabetes mellitus (IDDM) with consumption of A1 and A2 milk in 20 countries. The correlations, similar to their previous study, were extremely high: for ischaemic heart disease and A1 cow milk proteins, 'r' equaled 0.92 ($p < 0.00001$); for Type 1 diabetes mellitus r equaled 0.76 ($p < 0.001$). These were amazingly high correlation values.

As explained in Chapter One, a correlation of 1.0 means a one hundred percent equivalent incidence of the two factors being compared, which *suggests* that the one *causes* the other … or is caused by the same factor. The measure of correlation is the 'correlation coefficient, 'r', and is a measure of the linear relationship between two variables. If the relationship between two variables is non-linear, meaning that the incidence of the one variable does not move consistently with changes in the other variable, then the r – value has no significance. In statistical analysis, a correlation of 0.76 is very high, and 0.92 is exceptionally high. However, we must always keep in mind that correlation does not prove causation.

Another statistical technique is to square the 'r' value to obtain the 'coefficient of determination' which tells us the percent of the data that is 'closest to the line of best fit'. An r^2 value of 0.85 means that 85% of the total variation between the two variables can be explained by the proposed association, and only 15% can possibly be explained by other factors. The 'r^2' values for the correlation of A1 milk with heart disease and diabetes in Elliott's and Laugessen's study was 0.58 and 0.85, respectively.

The p-values calculated by Laugesen and Elliott are also significant. The p-value is the probability of obtaining a test statistic at least as extreme as the one that was actually observed. A p–value of 0.001 (one in a thousand chance) is the accepted norm for a credible association, which is what was derived for the diabetes association. And $p = 0.00001$ (one in a one-hundred-thousand chance), derived for the heart disease association, is considered exceptional. The strength of association found in the 2003 Laugessen and Elliott study is remarkable, and if not refuted, is by itself reason to take notice. Their work has been criticized, yes, and confounders have been proposed ... but the credibility of their work remains high ... *very* high !!

Corran McLachlan ... the heart disease connection

The story continues ... for the years 2000 through 2006 I rely heavily on Keith Woodford and his remarkable book, *Devil In The Milk*. During this period additional scientific study supporting the BCM-7 hypothesis was published, A2 Corportation was conceived and formed, Fonterra took over as the New Zealand dairy industry leader, and the 'great debate' emerged.

Corran McLachlan was a rare individual. As Woodford describes him, "He was one of those few people who could cross disciplines and make the great leaps needed to advance our understanding about the world we live in. He was also a man of great passion. But he was also a person who could work away painstakingly, putting together the detailed analyses on which the great leaps in knowledge are built." (pp 21) His achievements make a long list, and include 'Head Boy' and 'Senior Athletic Champion' at Wairarapa College, N.Z.; a first class honors degree in Chemical Engineering at Cambridge University, England; was the recipient of the first United Development Corporation Inventor's Prize in 1974; was General Manager at New Investments; Executive Director of Duncan & Davies Nurseries Ltd., and finally Managing Director of Tenon Development Ltd. McLachlan authored 29 scientific papers and confidential reports and holds 11 patents.

In the year 1994 Corran McLachlan was asked by the New Zealand Child Health Research Foundation to review Robert Elliott's research program. At that time McLachlan had been working on processes to manufacture low-cholesterol and cholesterol-free foods. McLachlan was struck by the similarity in Elliott's data and that which he had encountered in his own work ... data concerning IDDM incidence rates, and death rates due to ischaemic heart disease. He became strongly convinced that Elliott was on the right track, and began his own research. The businessman part in him also urged him to seek out how this new evidence could be put to use to make money.

In 2001 he published a meta-analysis study in the journal Medical Hypotheses entitled *Beta-casein A1, ischaemic heart disease mortality, and other illnesses*. The study used data from the World Health Organization (WHO) MONICA project and compared the incidence of ischaemic heart disease with the consumption of type A1 milk.

The "Multinational Monitoring of Trends and Determinants in Cardiovascular Disease Project", known as the MONICA Project, was established in the early 1980s in a number of centers around the world to monitor trends in cardiovascular diseases, and to relate these to changes in risk factors in the populations over a ten year period. There were a total of 32 MONICA Collaborating Centers located in 21 countries. The total number of men and women monitored, aged 25-84 years of age, exceeded ten million. The results were tabulated and published in the late 1990s, and the data are still being used for analysis even today.

McLachlan calculated that the correlation between ischaemic heart disease mortality and the consumption of type A1 milk was $r = 0.927$, and $r^2 = 0.86$. This calculation was similar to that concluded in the 1999 study by Elliott et al, and again the study by Elliott and Laugesen in 2003.

McLachlan also compared the incidence among the specific populations of Toulouse, France and Belfast, Ireland. The MONICA data showed that these two populations were almost identical in collective risk factors traditionally identified for heart disease. However, the consumption of type A1 milk in Belfast was 3.23 times that in Tolouse, *and* the heart disease mortality rate in Belfast was similarly just over three times that of Toulouse.

Including data about Type 1 diabetes, McLachlan was also able to show that the incidence of this disease closely matched with that of ischaemic heart disease in the populations studied, thus suggesting that the two disease conditions shared a common causative factor.

McLachlan also discussed the paradox of a very high consumption of cow's milk among the Masai and Samburu people of Kenya, who, surprisingly, have a very low incidence of heart disease ... it was known that the dairy cattle of these peoples produces only A2 milk. The Finland and French paradox was also revealed: The Fins are one of the highest per capita consumers of cow's milk in the world, and also with almost the highest incidence of heart disease ... the French consume a high per capita amount of cow's milk as well, yet their incidence of heart disease is much lower than in Finland. The milk consumed in Finland is from almost exclusively A1 cows, while the 'Normande' French breed produces close to pure A2. His observations and suggested conclusions were supported with statistics and graphical analysis.

In March, 2003, he published a letter in the New Zealand Medical Journal entitled *Setting the record straight: A1 β-casein, heart disease and diabetes*, which defended his 1999 study and went on to summarize additional statistical data demonstrating the strong epidemiological correlation between Type 1 diabetes and ischaemic heart disease mortality, emphasizing that a common factor was at play, and that this link could be the consumption of type A1 milk.

Although McLachlan was recognized for authoring these two valuable publications, his main contribution regarding the A1/A2 hypothesis was his influence in conveying the relevant science and data to the N.Z. Dairy Board and the N.Z. Dairy Research Institute. McLachlan was convinced that A1 beta-casein, and the BCM-7 peptide derived from it, comprised a major public health issue.

In Feberuary, 2000, McLachlan joined with New Zealand entrepreneur Howard Paterson to form a company named A2 Corporation. The concept was to commercialize the marketing of A2 milk by way of franchising and forming agreements with milk processors and marketers. This included copyrighting 'A2 Milk' as A2 Corporation's own brand, and patenting procedures to test dairy herds and milk samples for A1 versus A2 properties. NZ$12.8 million in capital was raised in the first year, with McLachlan assuming the position of Chief Executive and owning 35% in return for his intellectual property.

The details of how this came to pass makes fascinating reading, and is part of Woodford's writing ... well worth reading.

BCM-7 and heart disease ... oxidation of LDL ??

Given that an A1 milk/autoimmune mechanism may be at play with diabetes, and the observed close correlation between the incidence of Type 1 diabetes and ischaemic heart disease, then the question arises:

"what, then, is the possible mechanism by which the devil in the milk can contribute to heart disease ??"

Ischaemic heart disease (IHD), or 'myocardial ischaemia' is a disease characterized by a reduced blood supply to the heart muscles, usually due to blockage in the arteries, such as by the formation of arterial 'plaque', or the build-up of fatty materials such as cholesterol. The resultant thickening of the arterial walls, also known as 'atherosclerosis' slows down or stops the passage of blood, leading to a 'starved' condition and cellular death in the affected muscles. In the case of the heart this causes failure of heart muscle function, or 'myocardial infarction' (heart attack).

Atherosclerosis is still not well understood, but there is a strong consensus that the oxidation of 'low-density-lipoprotein' (LDL) is a key factor. It may act via oxidized LDL to damage arterial walls and then to become part of the actual plaque build-up, or it may simply be the material used in the build-up. With either scenario, this is where BCM-7 enters the scene ... BCM-7 is known to be a strong oxidant.

Once again there is a paucity of supportive studies, and there are a number of articles and studies which attempt to refute the premise that the BCM-7 peptide may be linked to LDL oxidation. Four supportive studies stand out: one by Torreilles et al in 1995, one by Tailford et al in 2003, and a pair of studies by Steinerova et al in 1999 and 2001. All four studies have been strongly criticized, and the Steinerova studies do not directly address the possible role of beta-casomorphins.

The study by the French scientist, Jean Torreilles, and his co-worker, Marie-Christian Guerin is by far the most directly supportive study. Titled *Casein-derived peptides can promote human LDL oxidation by a perosidase-dependent and metal-dependent process,* they were able to demonstrate under laboratory conditions that the 'tyrosyl radical' (a free radical, generated by damaged tyrosine amino acid) could act as a catalyst to oxidize LDL lipids. (Torrielles, 1995) Their work has been much discussed, but not refuted.

Tailford et al (Julie Campbell was the leader and corresponding author) took this a step further with their study in 2002, using rabbits as test animals. They were able to show that rabbits fed type A1 beta-casein developed fatty plaque lesions that were both larger and thicker than those of rabbits fed A2 beta-casein. Unfortunately, they were not able to demonstrate that the correlation was statistically significant, and the study was further criticized because it was commissioned by A2 Corporation.

189

Again there is a great need for high-quality, credible studies. Never-the-less, the Torreilles and Tailford studies, even by themselves, do give credible evidence that the BCM-7 peptide is a strong oxidant, and *does* have the capability to oxidize LDL cholesterol.

The opiate BCM-7 ... the connection with autism, schizophrenia, and other neurological disorders

The proposed link between autism, schizophrenia, and other neurological diseases with gluten (wheat protein) and casein (milk protein) has been around for a long time. The treatment by consuming a diet free of these two proteins ... named the 'gluten-free, casein-free (GFCF) diet ... has been tried by a large number of individuals over more than four decades, with a very long list of positive testimonials.

One of the first to connect autism and schizophrenia with diet was Dr. Curtis Dothan in the early 1960s. He identified the first phenomena that suggested the linkage, which was the observation that schizophrenic sufferers very often had unusually permeable digestive systems and digested both the gluten protein from wheat and the casein protein from milk inefficiently (upon digestion, the protein failed to break down completely to individual amino acids). Dr. Jaak Panksepp reported the same observations in 1979.

The theory was given new insight when Dr. Kalle Reichelt found that gluten and casein peptides were commonly present in the urine of autistic children, but not in the urine of normal children. Reichelt went on to be the first to suggest that upon digestion by autistic sufferes, the proteins were not broken down successfully or completely into individual amino acids, but instead allowed some fragments, or peptides, to break away intact, and these peptides could then pass through abnormally permeable stomach or intestinal linings. This phenomenon is once again our 'leaky gut' scenario. However, it is important to note that in the autistic or schizophrenic what may be critical is the combination of inefficient digestion of the proteins on one hand, with a permeable, or 'leaky gut' on the other. The theorized passage of protein peptides and presence in the blood stream is a result of, first, incomplete digestion into individual amino acids, and secondly, the ability of the larger peptide fragments to pass through a leaky gut.

Now, this explains how a peptide or beta-casomorphin can enter the body. However, if the peptide is causally associated with neurological dysfunction, they must be able to enter the brain. However, our designers gave us a marvelous gift to prevent damage to that most crucial part of our body ... the *blood-brain barrier*. Abbreviated BBB, the blood-brain barrier is a separation of circulating blood and cerebral fluid ... the fluid that our brain literally 'floats' in. The barrier occurs along all blood capillaries going to the brain and consists of tight junctions that are unique to only that area. 'Endothelial cells' restrict the passage of microscopic objects such as bacteria and larger 'hydrophilic' molecules (are non-soluble in water), yet allow 'hydrophobic' (water-soluble) molecules to pass. These hydrophobic molecules include hormones and oxygen. Certain cells of the barrier also actively transport minerals, glucose, and other compounds via specific barrier proteins.

So ... the question is then asked: "Can the opioid peptides such as BCM-7 (and gliadorphin) cross the blood-brain barrier? In 1999 Drs Robert Cade and Zhongjie Sun et al completed a study with rats that demonstrated conclusively that yes, the BCM-7 beta-casomorphin can pass through the blood-brain barrier. (Sun et al, 1999).

Thus one more piece to the puzzle was put in place.

It is also crucial to understand that the peptides from wheat gluten can be very similar to those derived from casein. I was surprised in my research to find that much of what we now know about gluten peptides is relatively new knowledge.

Our cereals grains, as we now know them, are a relatively new food for us humans. Similar to the case of cow's milk, we did not domesticate cereal grains such as wheat until about 9,000 years ago ... perhaps 2,000 years before we domesticated *Bos taurus*, the cow. This has been suggested to be one reason why we have trouble with cereal proteins ... our physiologies may simply not be designed for this come-along-lately food.

The nutritional value of the grains make them an important food choice, however. One hundred grams of hard red winter wheat, for example, contains about 71 grams of carbohydrate, 1.5 g of total fat, 12.2 g of dietary fiber, and 12.6 grams of protein, and is an important source for many vitamins and minerals, notably iron. The main protein is 'gluten' which comprises about 80% of the protein in wheat. It is also the main protein in rye and barley.

Gluten is the composite of two proteins, named *gliadin* and *glutenin*. It is important to note that, although the protein in maize and rice are sometimes called gluten, they do not contain the gliadin portion. Gliadin, similar to casein, can separate into peptide fragments, and these peptides

191

can also have opiate properties. The most significant is the seven amino acid chain called *gliadorphin,* or *gluteomorphin.* Yes … a 7-amino acid fragment !! The amino-acid sequence is Tyr-Pro-Gly-Pro-Gly-Pro-Phe (using the abbreviated forms). Surprisingly, this plant source peptide compares very closely to the animal-derived beta-casomorphin (BCM-7): Tyr-Pro-Phe-Pro-Gly-Pro-Ile. Notably, both peptides begin with a tyrosine followed by a proline, have a glycine or phenylalanine in the third location, and both have a total of 3 prolines each. Both gliadorphin and BCM-7 are therefore strong opiates, and are very stable. And, as Woodford points out, the two morphin peptides 'hunt together'.

The four scientists that stand out in this special field of inquiry are Robert Cade, Zhongjie Sun, Paul Shattock, and Kalle Reichelt. Cade and Sun were researchers at the University of Florida, Shattock was from the Autism Research Unit at the University of Sunderland, and Reichelt was from the Pediatrics Research Institute at the University of Oslo. Dr. Cade, who is famous as the inventor of 'Gatorade', died on November 16th, 2007 … much of his work has been carried on by his colleague, Dr. Sun.

These three groups have interacted together, and a number of their studies have been published in the journals Nutritional Neuroscience, Autism, and Brain Dysfunction. The key concept underlining their work is that many of the symptoms of neurological dysfunction are related to what we eat and how we metabolize what we eat. Particular foods that they have targeted include the two proteins, gluten and casein, and the opioid peptides that these two proteins are able to generate. They have shown that residues of gliadorphin and BCM-7 consistently show up in the urine of autistic children. They also report remarkable success with diets that are free of gluten and casein.

One intriguing piece of support to the BCM-7 association with neurological disorders was presented by none other than the New Zealand Dairy Board. By way of some in-depth investigation and probing, Woodford was able to retrieve their application for a patent to supply A2 milk, presented in 2001. The application was entitled *Milk containing beta-casein with proline at position 67 does not aggravate neurological disorders.* The wording of this application is critical to the over-all credibility of the entire A1/A2 hypothesis, and sheds light on the mischievous switch by Fonterra later on to disavow the same hypothesis. Keep in mind that the Dairy Board, in essence, became Fonterra, and the same people were the key players then and afterwards. For example, Jeremy Hill was a co-author, and later became the 'Chief of Technology'. I have therefore included the abstract in whole:

'The invention is based on the discovery that the consumption of milk which contains a beta-casein-variant which has histidine or any other amino acid not proline at position 67, may on digestion cause the release of an opioid which may induce or aggravate a neurological/mental disorder such as autism or Asperger's syndrome. The invention is supplying milk or milk products that contain beta-casein with proline at position 67 to susceptible individuals." (*Devil In The Milk*, pp 135)

How do opioid beta-casomorphins promote disease conditions ??

So ... how do opiates contribute to disease conditions ?? Wang et al, in their 2008 paper entitled *Opiate abuse, innate immunity, and bacterial infectious diseases,* explains that opiates can damage immune defenses that are essential for carrying out rapid immune reactions to invading pathogens. They state that "in vitro studies with innate immune cells from experimental animals and humans and in vivo studies with animal models have shown that opiate abuse impairs innate immunity and is responsible for increased susceptibility to bacterial infection." (Wang et al, 2008).

A number of other recent studies have suggested associations with opiate consumption and a variety of disease conditions. Noel et al (2008) reviews the effects of opiates on the immune system and its effect on HIV replication and the progress of AIDS. Howard et al (2010) finds evidence to indicate that opiate use among women with or at risk for HIV is associated with increased risk for diabetes.

Research has also implicated the BCM-7 molecule in impaired learning of infants and young children. Dubynin et al (2008) tested the effect of several opioid peptides on the learning ability of albino rat pups, and found that the BCM-7 peptide had a significant negative effect.

A recent Russian study by Kost et al (Kost, 2009) found that babies fed with cow's milk based formula containing BCM-7 demonstrated significant delay in psychomotor development.

Unfortunately, I have been unable to find any additional high-quality trials (i.e., double-blind trials) investigating the possible connection of type A1 or type A2 milk specifically with autism or other neurological disorders, and there is now an apparent lack of continued interest in this line of study ... or perhaps a lack of funding. Even Sun, Shattock, and Reichelt seem to have lost interest. There is a great need for credible, double-blinded studies to be undertaken.

Milk allergy, milk intolerance, celiac disease, Crohn's disease, ulcerative colitis, sudden-death-syndrome, multiple sclerosis, and Parkinson's disease

Keith Woodford, in *Devil In The Milk*, explores the possible connection of BCM-7 and other beta-casomorphins with a number of additional disease conditions. He examines each in detail, and his statements and conclusions are compelling. However, what we now know about the possible link of beta-casomorphins, particularly BCM-7, with disease conditions such as milk allergy, milk intolerance, celiac disease, Crohn's disease, ulcerative colitis, sudden-death-syndrome, multiple sclerosis, and Parkinson's disease is sketchy, and highly conjectural. Some of these conditions relate to the condition of a 'leaky gut', and are therefore associated more with the process of how beta-casomorphins can enter the body that with their effect once in the body. Some conditions suggest that an auto-immune response is involved. Others that an oxidative process is at play. Or that an unknown neurological dysfunction in the brain is related, possibly caused by the strong opiate property of the beta-casomorphins.

Keith Woodford suggests that we take the BCM-7 hypothesis seriously, and consider the 'big picture':

"What we do know for sure is that for each disease there is one or more environmental trigger. We also know that milk keeps coming up as a prime candidate. If milk contains the cause then it almost certainly has to be one or more bioactive proteins in the milk. It is also likely that opioids are involved. It is hard to go past BCM-7 as a likely candidate. ... Undoubtedly there will be false leads, and the answers will be complex. It seems to me that BCM-7 is leaving enough tell-tale signs that it is eventually going to be unmasked as a villain. Surely it would be better that our milk was free of this devil." (pp 158)

2. Fonterra

New Zealand is truly a 'land of milk and honey'! Annual production of honey exceeds 11,000 tons ... with a population of only 4.2 million, that equals about 4 pounds per capita per year. And how about milk? ... Well, New Zealand is the home of one dairy cow for each man, woman, and child in the country, and produces over 15 million tons of milk per year ...

194

or about 3.6 tons per person. Dairy is New Zealand's largest industry and biggest export earner.

The dairy industry in New Zealand has traditionally been characterized by a large number of individual dairy farms, usually small family-owned operations, which join collectively in co-ops to market their product. Prior to 2001 the N.Z. farmers were united under the New Zealand Dairy Board, with all but a very few of the dairy farms in the nation joined in one marketing cooperative. But the decision to deregulate in that year resulted in the formation of Fonterra Cooperative Group Ltd., with 10,500 individual farms, or 95% of the total N.Z. farms. Westland Co-operative Dairy Company and Tatua Cooperative Dairy Company Ltd. elected not to join Fonterra, and made up the remaining 5%.

Fonterra has been a success story, expanding rapidly since 2001, and has now become a major player in the global dairy industry. The latest statistics rank Fonterra as the fifth largest dairy company in the world ... and the largest milk processor. Ninety-five percent of New Zealand's milk and milk product production is exported. This amount significantly affects the total global picture ... while New Zealand's milk production accounts for only 2% of world production, it accounts for 33% of world trade in dairy products. Key products include cheeses, protein concentrates, and biomedical and biohealth products. It is estimated that Fonterra currently controls as much as 40% of the world's dairy industry.

Fonterra and A1, A2 milk

Before deregulation in 2001, and for some time afterwards, the N.Z. mainstream dairy industry was keenly interested in the A1/A2 hypothesis. This was largely due to the studies by Robert Elliot and Jeremy Hill, and the influence of Corran McLachlan. For example, the New Zealand Dairy Board was a co-applicant on a patent which cited an association of type A1 milk with diabetes (2000), and another one which cited an association with autism (2001). Jeremy Hill was then with the Dairy Board's research arm, the New Zealand Dairy Research Institute, and authored reports to support the patent applications. A copy of one of these reports was given to Howard Paterson (A2 Corporation). In this report Jeremy Hill acknowleged the science and data in support of the A1/A2 hypothesis, and included some research of his own. When Fonterra was formed Dr. Hill became Group Director of Technology for Fonterra's equivalence to the NZDRI, called the Fonterra Research Centre. In 2006 Jeremy Hill was also co-author of an Icelandic study which linked A1 milk consumption and type 1 diabetes (reviewed above).

There was even a program underway to convert New Zealand dairy herds to A2 producers. By 2001 the New Zealand Dairy Board, which also administered the national dairy cattle breeding system, had decided to test the A1/A2 status of all the dairy bulls. There was a strong interest in the conversion. Woodford reports that as of 2005 approximately 500 N.Z. farmers were in the process of converting to A2 milk.

Prior to the year 2005 Fonterra sought patents similar to, and in competition with those being applied for by A2 Corporation. On July 4th, 2005, the Intellectual Property Office of New Zealand ruled against Fonterra and in favor of A2 Corporation on all matters pertaining to the patent applications by both companies.

3. The 'great debate'

It is not clear just when the New Zealand Dairy Board first decided to stand up against A2 Corporation, but Woodford suggests that it was probably soon after the fateful meeting in October, 2000, between Howard Patterson of A2 Corporation and Warren Larson, N.Z. Dairy Board Chief. Woodford reports:

> "It was at that meeting that phrases like 'class-action' started to be thrown about by Howard Paterson in relation to non-disclosure of key information. Warren Larsen was clearly concerned that A2 Corporation was a bunch of irresponsible cowboys that could put the New Zealand dairy industry at risk. They needed to be stopped in their tracks."

After the takeover by Fonterra, the animosity and competitiveness between Fonterra and A2 Corporation intensified. It was a curious situation. At that time Fonterra was supportive of the A1/A2 hypothesis and was interested in obtaining the same sort of patents and copyrights as did A2 Corporation. But the competitiveness over patents intensified, and outright animosity became the prevailing mood. The deaths of both Paterson and McLachlan in 2003 surely added to Fonterra's confidence that they would succeed over A2 Corporation in all aspects. The ruling by the Intellectual Property Office in favor of A2 Corporation in 2005 must have been a severe blow to Fonterra, and a turning point. From then on they were not only against A2 Corporation, but were against the entire A1/A2 hypothesis.

The ensuing debate is full of intrigue, mischievous and outright unethical science, plus the muscling of big business.

A key factor was clearly the untimely deaths of both Howard Paterson and Corran McLachland in 2003. Conspiracy advocates have jumped to the sensationalist conclusion that their deaths were programmed by other interests, but Woodford reports otherwise. Howard Paterson was in Fiji on July 1, 2003 for a business meeting, but failed to show up. He was found dead in his hotel room, and the autopsy determined that he had, in fact, choked on some potato chips. He was 50 years old. Corran McLachlan had been fighting a losing battle with melanoma cancer for ten years, and died early in August, also 2003. He was 59.

The deaths of these two men could have meant the end of A2 Corporation, and the A1/A2 milk issue may have died with them. Indeed, the ensuing effort by Fonterra, which took the place of the New Zealand Dairy Board, was aimed in that direction. The next segment of the unfolding story, again related by Woodford, is about Fonterra's counter attack and subsequent articles and studies that attempted to negate the A1/A2 hypothesis. It is again absorbing reading. Once more, I encourage the reader to read *Devil In The Milk*. For this part Dr. Woodford is not only a writer and a reporter, but is an investigating journalist and a scientist.

The pros

The case for the A1/A2 milk (BCM-7) hypothesis begins and ends with the scientific evidence, with perhaps an additional touch of logical inference. In summary, the evidence supporting the hypothesis can be divided into 11 different arguments:

1. The epidemiological evidence that demonstrates a remarkably high correlation between consumption of A1 versus A2 milk and the incidence of both type 1 diabetes (IDDM) and ischaemic heart disease (IHD). The studies by Elliott and McLachlan stand out is this respect. The more specific comparisons of the populations of Finland versus France and Iceland, the Samoan children living in New Zealand versus their home country, and the Masai and Samburu people of Kenya, each add compelling examples.

2. The fact that BCM-7 is generated only from A1 beta-casein ... A1 and A2 beta-casein are digested differently because of the histidine at position 67 instead of a proline, and therefore generate very different peptides, with very different properties.

3. The fact that BCM-7 caso-morphin can enter the body (a) under permeable stomach and small intestine lining conditions (ie. infants), (b) or under 'leaky gut' conditions, (c) plus evidence that it can enter even under normal conditions either after truncation by the enzyme 'dipeptidyl peptidase 4' (DPP4), located on the intestine lining, or at the position known as Caco-2 on the intestinal lining.

4. The fact that the BCM-7 peptide is an opioid beta-casomorphin, is a strong oxidant, and the amino acid composition is identical in the final four positions to the GLUT 2 molecule in the pancreas beta-cell. Each of these properties help explain the promotion of specific disease conditions.

5. The finding that mice and rats fed A1 beta-casein have a higher incidence of Type 1 diabetes (IDDM).

6. Evidence that rabbits fed on alternate diets of A1 versus A2 milk developed greater accumulations of arterial plaque within the aorta artery (atherosclerosis).

7. The evidence that autistic and schizophrenic children typically excrete large amount of BCM-7 in their urine, whereas normal children do not.

8. Identification of specific mechanisms whereby BCM-7 can (a) promote an auto-immune attack on pancreas beta-cells, (b) act as a strong oxidant on LDL, and (c) can pass through the blood-brain barrier and act as an opioid to promote neurological dysfunction.

9. The evidence that autistic and schizophrenic children typically excrete large amount of BCM-7 in their urine, whereas normal children do not.

10. The finding that persons with certain disease conditions often and consistently contain antibodies for BCM-7 in their bloodstream.

11. The extensive anecdotal evidence (testimonials) from persons who have switched to A2 milk and report improvements in a number of disease conditions.

The counter-attack

The basic stance that the New Zealand Dairy Board, and later Fonterra, decided to take on the type A1 beta-casein issue was evident as far back as 1997. Even back then there was enough information and concern circulating among board members to warrant a group-wide decision. They needed to decide on whether or not to initiate breeding techniques to switch New Zealand's dairy herds from mainly type A1 milk producers to type A2 producers. Keith Woodford explains that he was able to obtain unpublished documents from the New Zealand Dairy Group (the largest dairy co-operative at that time) and the New Zealand Dairy Research Institute (NZDRI) related to the industry's discussions. He reports this information in his paper to the International Diabetes Federation (IDF) Congress, in 2008. The documents reveal that it was a close decision for them. The challenge at hand would be first to convert the herds, which could be a ten-year process or more, and secondly the problem of how to protect the market for the continuing A1 milk being produced, and to create a new market for the new type A2 milk. The challenge, and the cost, would be formidable. The decision by the NZ Dairy Board was to do nothing overt, especially not to cause concern among the public, and to hope that the issue would fade away. (Woodford, 2008)

But with the published studies by Elliott and Laugesen, and McLachlan, the issue did not fade away. And then A2 Corporation was formed. Now re-organized as Fonterra, the NZ Dairy Board was at first open to the A1/A2 issue, and took a positive stance. They even sought after the same sort of patents that A2 Corporation was seeking, that would give them a marketing edge, and wrote reports to support the A1/A2 milk (BCM-7) hypothesis. But this attitude and strategy changed over time with an increasing competitiveness and growing animosity between Fonterra and A2 Corporation, and then with the ruling by the Intellectual Property Office of New Zealand on July 4th, 2005 'in favor of A2 Corporation on all matters pertaining to the patent applications by both companies'.

The FAD trial

In 2001 the New Zealand Dairy Board took the initiative to sponsor a large-scale international study to expand on Elliot's earlier work with rats and mice, to further test the association of A1 β-casein with diabetes. It is not clear whether the NZ Dairy Board was supportive of the A1/A2 milk (BCM-7) hypothesis in undertaking this study, or that they changed their position somewhere enroute. Never-the-less, the published results were highly negative.

The study was entitled *A multi-centre, blinded international trial of the effect of A1 and A2 β-casein variants on diabetes incidence in two rodent models of spontaneous Type 1 diabetes,* and was authored by nine scientists. Three of them are already known to this discussion: Robert Elliott, Jeremy Hill, and P. Pozzilli. The others were P.E Beales, R.B. Flohe', H. Kolb, G.S. Wang, H. Wasmuth, and F.W. Scott. Because

Beales was the first author named, the study has sometimes been called the Beales et al study. But Frazer Scott was the listed 'corresponding author' and is therefore assumed to be the team leader. As a whole the nine authors represented New Zealand, Canada, Great Britain, Germany, and Italy.

Three laboratories were set up: one in New Zealand, one in Canada, and one in Great Britain. Two rodent species were used: the BB mice, and the NOD rat, which are both known to be susceptible to diabetes. From the very beginning, the study had many flaws. The rodent species were not consistent, and the diets were complicated: four were based on a casein-based product called 'Pregestimil', four were based on a soy bean product called 'Prosobee', and one of the diets was a milk-free, cereal-based rodent diet. Both the Pregestimil and the Prosobee are human infant formulas produced and marketed by Mead Johnson. All the diets were prepared in New Zealand and distributed from there.

The study then encountered a series of problems. First, the New Zealand mice suffered from an outbreak of 'Clostridium disease' and many died. The New Zealand trial portion was therefore abandoned. This lab was under the supervision of Robert Elliott, who then stood back as a primary player. The second calamity was that the Pregetimil used was found to already have a high content of BCM-7. This fact was reported by Jeremy Hill in a document dated October, 2000. However, no mention of this was made in the final paper published in the journal Diabetologia in 2002, and it is not clear whether all the authors were aware of this fact. The importance of this is tantamount to invalidating the entire trial … it meant that a strong confounder was present, and the data would also be invalid.

Woodford one again was the relentless pursuer, and he contacted the various authors, scrutinized the data, and even went to battle with the journal, Diabetologia. Robert Elliot reported that he was not aware of this event, and made the following statement in an email to Woodford:

"I am still upset by this news. Why did Jeremy do that?? If the Pregestimil used contained BCM-7 when the manufacturers state that no peptide (more than) 4 amino acids in length is present in their product, something odd has happened.

It of course invalidates the Pregestimil arm of the FAD study. This means that the two major conclusions of the FAD study are invalid." (*Devil In The Milk,* pp 106-7)

A great deal of cover-up, denials of responsibility, and a refusal to retract the study from Diabetologia ensued. Jeremy Hill denied that he had known about the Pregestimil contamination. Diabetologia even refused to investigate, or to print an acknowledgement that the study had been flawed. In a final heated communication with the editor, Woodford referred him to a much quoted editorial from the December, 2005 issue of New Scientist:

"Science runs on trust. Governments give researchers money on the understanding they will use it fairly and honestly report their results. Peer reviewers assume that what they are judging is a fair account of what happened; they are not yet charged with policing dubious data. Without trust the whole scientific world will collapse." (*Devil In The Milk*, pp 114)

It is interesting that Robert Elliot later joined with Keith Woodford in various communications and media presentations, and has consistently supported the A1/A2 milk (BCM-7) hypothesis, and has stated repeatedly that the FAD trial was flawed and the conclusions invalid. In addition, Woodford re-analyzed the FAD data, correcting for the contaminated Pregetimil, and concludes that the data do, in fact, support the correlation between consumption of type A1 beta-casein and an increased incidence of Type 1 diabetes.

Fraser Scott and Hubert Kolb, two of the FAD trial authors, later published a review entitled *A1 β-casein milk and Type 1 diabetes: causal relationship probed in animal models* in The New Zealand Medical Journal, March 2003. They repeated the same data and conclusions as the flawed FAD trial ... and of course they failed to mention that the Pregetimil feed was contaminated with BCM-7.

Fonterra paper, 2004

Early in 2004 Fonterra, even before the ruling of the Intellectual Property Office, began their counter-attack. A 12-page document was released (but never published) that set the groundwork for their assault. Woodford reports that this report "included many erroneous statements, and a number of quotes taken seriously out of context." (Woodford, 2008)

The New Zealand Food Safety Authority (NZFSA), and the Swinburn report

According to their website, the "New Zealand Food Safety Authority's mandate is to protect consumers by providing an effective food regulatory programme covering food produced and consumed in New Zealand as well as imports and exports of food products". Its two-fold task is the protection and promotion of public health and safety, and the promotion and facilitation of access to markets for New Zealand food and food products. In the past the agency worked closely with the New Zealand Ministry of Agriculture and Forestry (MAF) … as of July, 2010 the New Zealand Food Safety Authority and MAF were joined as a single government regulation and monitoring agency.

Within days after the publication of Elliott and Laugesen's study in January, 2003, the NZFSA issued a press release entitled *Milk Still Part of Balanced Diet*. The release acknowledged Elliott and Laugesen's finding, but concluded:

"The Ministry of Health supports the NZFSA's view that the evidence is not strong enough to change the health messages around milk or to require any special labeling on milk or milk products … milk is nutritious and beneficial and should remain part of a balanced diet." (*Devil In The Milk*, pp 169)

By March, 2003, NZFSA was in negotiation with Dr. Boyd Swinburn from Deakin University in Australia to review the A1/A2 milk (BCM-7) hypothesis and to author a report. Swinburn was also the former Medical Director of the National Heart Foundation of New Zealand. Swinburn drafted his report within a couple of months, but the report was not released until August, 2004. There was a great deal of inside debate going on during this period, which Woodford reports and discusses in *Devil In The Milk*. Just before his death, Corran McLachlan was also involved, and Woodford reports that he was furious with NZFSA's decision to seek out a review study by Swinburn.

With publication of the report, NZFSA issued its own press release, stating:

"There is no food safety issue with either type of milk … Professor Swinburn's review show that there is insufficient evidence to demonstrate benefits of one type of milk protein over another."

However, there was definitely some mischief at play. When NZFSA released Swinburn's report for publication, it was discovered that omissions and changes had been made to the report. First of all, the 'Lay

Summary' had been left out, which contained some conclusions that were contradictory to NZFSA's released statements. Plus, the length of the document had been 'stretched' by inserting extra spaces between paragraphs in an attempt to conceal the fact that omissions had been made. Interestingly, since the time of publication back in 2004, Keith Woodford has had numerous communications and meetings with Dr. Swinburn, and Dr. Swinburn has joined with Woodford in media presentations and written statements ... he is actually very supportive of the A1/A2 milk (BCM-7) hypothesis, and is dismayed that the NZFSA has mis-represented his conclusions.

With heavy pressure from the media and Woodford, with Woodford being the prime motivator, the Lay Summary was finally released, and NZFSA even put it on its website ... but the damage had been done, and the news was already old. Never-the-less, what the Lay Summary actually said is important, and so I am including the final three paragraphs (from *Devil In The Milk,* pp 174-5):

"The A1/A2 hypothesis is both intriguing and potentially very important for public health if it is proved correct. It should be taken seriously and further research is needed. In addition, the appropriate government agencies have a responsibility to communicate the current state of evidence to the public, including uncertainty about the evidence. Further public health actions, such as changing dietary advice or requiring labeling of milk products, are not considered to be warranted at this stage. Monitoring is also required to ensure that any claims made for A2 milk fall within the regulations for food claims.

Changing the dairy herds to more A2 producing cows is an option for the dairy and associated industries and these decisions will undoubtedly be made on a commercial basis. Changing dairy herds to more A2 producing cows may significantly improve public health, if the A1/A2 hypothesis is proved correct, and it is highly unlikely to do harm.

As a matter of individual choice, people may wish to reduce or remove A1 beta-casein from their diet (or their children's diet) as a precautionary measure. This may be particularly relevant for those individuals who have or are at risk of the diseases mentioned (Type 1 diabetes, coronary heart disease, autism and schizophrenia). However, they should do so knowing that there is substantial uncertainty about the benefits of such an approach."

Woodford tells us that Dr. Swinburn had argued with the NZFSA, including telling them in one communication that:

"… if I had a child with Type 1 diabetes and was due to have another and I could easily obtain and afford A2 milk or formula, I would certainly use it for the next child because the cost/benefit is low because of the potentially very large benefit of preventing Type 1 diabetes."

A copy of the Lay Summary to the report is now available online from the NZFSA website: www.nzfsa.govt.nz/policy-law/projects/a1-a2-milk/lay-summary.htm

A.S. Truswell; *The A2 milk case: a critical review*

This review was published in the European Journal of Clinical Nutrition, in November, 2005. It has been cited extensively by agencies and other scientists interested in discrediting the A1/A2 milk (BCM-7) hypothesis. It is worthwhile to present the entire abstract to the study, which is as follows:

"This review outlines a hypothesis that A1 one of the common variants of β-casein, a major protein in cow's milk could facilitate the immunological processes that lead to type 1 diabetes (DM-1). It was subsequently suggested that A1 β-casein may also be a risk factor for coronary heart disease (CHD), based on between-country correlations of CHD mortality with estimated national consumption of A1 β-casein in a selected number of developed countries. A company, A2 Corporation was set up in New Zealand in the late 1990s to test cows and market milk in several countries with only the A2 variant of β-casein, which appeared not to have the disadvantages of A1 β-casein.

The second part of this review is a critique of the A1/A2 hypothesis. For both DM-1 and CHD, the between-country correlation method is known to be unreliable and negated by recalculation with more countries and by prospective studies in individuals. The animal experiments with diabetes-prone rodents that supported the hypothesis about diabetes were not confirmed by larger, better standardized multicentre experiments. The single animal experiment supporting an A1 β-casein and CHD link was small, short, in an unsuitable animal model and had other design weaknesses.

The A1/A2 milk hypothesis was ingenious. If the scientific evidence had worked out it would have required huge adjustments in the world's dairy industries. This review concludes, however, that there is no convincing or even probable evidence that the A1 β-casein of cow milk has any adverse effect in humans.

204

This review has been independent of examination of evidence related to A1 and A2 milk by the Australian and New Zealand food standard and food safety authorities, which have not published the evidence they have examined and the analysis of it. They stated in 2003 that no relationship has been established between A1 or A2 milk and diabetes, CHD or other diseases." (Truswell, 2004)

Woodford devotes several pages in *Devil In The Milk* to answering Truswell's criticisms, and I think his effort is convincing. It is lengthy and in-depth ... I recommend that the reader go through it. Truswell chose to resort to a number of arguments which erroneously reported and interpreted data, were not even logical in places, and he did not present any convincing counter-evidence of his own. No conflicting data was offered.

His main three counter-arguments centered on (a) epidemiological studies and data do not establish proof, (b) that Elliott's prior mice and rat studies were invalidated by the larger, higher quality FAD trial, and (c) that rabbits were are inappopriate model for studying atherosclerosis. Well, we already know that correlation does not establish proof, and in fact, final proof is a very elusive element in science. As for the FAD trial, we know that it was seriously flawed and the conclusions invalid. About using rabbits as test animals?? ... it is a common, accepted model for a great deal of research of this type.

The tone of his paper is clearly negative, even resorting to the implication that the A1/A2 hypothesis was all an 'ingenious scheme'.

However, the axe that gives the final blow to Truswell's attempted expose' is that it was discovered later that he was under hire by Fonterra at the time ... Woodford's relentless and persistent investigation revealed that he was being employed by Fonterra as their 'key external scientific witness' in the 2004/2005 hearings with the New Zealand Intellectual Property Office, in which Fonterra ending up losing in all matters to A2 Corporation. Now this is truly an interesting scenario: Truswell was Fonterra's key witness in efforts to secure patents that would give them intellectual property rights and a marketing edge in promoting A2 milk (and the A1/A2 hypothesis) ... but then, after this legal battle was lost in full to A2 Corporation in the month of July, 2005, Truswell then went on to author a review attempting to trash the entire A1/A2 hypothesis four months later. The word 'trash' is appropriate in this respect ... both as the verb and then as the noun.

NZFSA update, October 10th, 2007

When *Devil In The Milk* was first published in New Zealand in September 2007 the response was immediate and extra-ordinare ... Woodford reports that he was interviewed through the radio and television media forty times in the first week. He explains that he heard nothing from Fonterra, except that they had contacted him just before publication, asking him to delay the publication for six months. The NZFSA, however "came out with all guns blazing".

The New Zealand Food Safety Authority published an update on October 10th, 2007 explaining that they were in communication with the European Food Safety Authority (EFSA) and confirmed that the EFSA was planning to review the possible health hazards of A1 β-casein-rich milk.

In the report, the NZFSA acknowledged Keith Woodford, and his book, *Devil In The Milk*, and the A1/A2 (BCM-7) hypothesis ... and also acknowledged the considerable media interest preceding and following the publication. The tentative NZFSA conclusion was:

"There is no scientific consensus on this hypothesis and material presented in the book is open to scientific debate."

For this reason, their position regarding the A1/A2 issue was summed up by the Minister of Food Safety, Honorable Lianne Dalziel, in the following statement:

"I consider that as EFSA is undertaking a comprehensive review of the existing science associated with A1 and A2 milk, a separate New Zealand review, as originally proposed by NZFSA in October 2007, will not be necessary." (Dalziel, 2008)

4. The EFSA Report

The home page of the EFSA website states their purpose and scope as follows:

"The European Food Safety Authority (EFSA) is the keystone of European Union (EU) risk assessment regarding food and feed safety. In close collaboration with national authorities and in open consultation with its stakeholders, EFSA provides independent scientific advice and clear communication on existing and emerging risks." (www.efsa.europa.eu/en/aboutefsa.htm)

The agency was established in January, 2002, with their head office in Parma, Italy. Their scope of responsibility extends to include animal health and welfare, and crop plant issues.

Their website goes on to say:

"EFSA's goal is to become globally recognized as the European reference body for risk assessment on food and feed safety, animal health and welfare, nutrition, plant protection and plant health. EFSA's independent scientific advice underpins the European food safety system. Thanks to this system, European consumers are among the best protected and best informed in the world as regards risks in the food chain."

This is heady wording ! One cannot help but be impressed, and in fact, confident that with this agency we are going to receive a fair and responsible assessment.

The New Zealand Food Safety Authority (NZFSA) met with the EFSA in December, 2007, requesting that the EFSA review the A1/A2 milk (BCM-7) hypothesis. The EFSA accepted. It was clear that the NZFSA held the EFSA in high esteem, positioning them as a 'higher authority', which was stated in their April 2nd, 2008 report:

"EFSA is a highly resourced, competent and internationally respected authority with a wealth of expertise in the areas of risk assessment and food safety."

With confirmation that the EFSA would undertake the review, the NZFSA added:

"I consider that as EFSA is undertaking a comprehensive review of the existing science associated with A1 and A2 milk, a separate New Zealand review, as originally proposed by NZFSA in October, 2007, will not be necessary." (Dalziel, 2008)

The NZFSA worked with the EFSA, and made available all the data and studies which they had themselves acquired, specifically including the Swinburn report (this was mentioned in the DalZiel report)

Their review is entitled *Review of the potential health impact of β-casomorphins and related peptides*, and is sub-titled a *Report of the DATEX Working Group on β-casomorphins*. The report was issued on January 29th, 2009. It took 13 months for them to complete the project, starting from when the New Zealand Food Safety Authority asked them to undertake the review in December, 2007. The report is 107 pages long.

However, 39 pages are devoted to listing an impressive number of references ... 535 of them, in fact. This is more than impressive ... it is many more than what I could find myself that are directly related to this issue ... and there may be a reason for this. I will explain in the ensuing paragraphs.

An aside: the 'Betacasein.net' website, which is devoted to compiling up-to-date scientific literature on the A1/A2 issue listed only 80 studies in their 2008 review.

The conclusion to the report is contained in a two-sentence finale' at the end of their summary, and is curiously repeated as the totality of their 'Recommendations' at the very end of the report:

"Based on the present review of available scientific literature, a cause-effect relationship between the oral intake of BCM-7 or related peptides and aetiology or course of any suggested non-communicable diseases cannot be established. Consequently, a formal EFSA risk assessment of food-derived peptides is not recommended."

This conclusion was probably predictable. Many, including Woodford, feel that it was. One has only to look at how the agency was tasked with the review, by whom, the studies specifically emphasized beforehand, and the conclusions already reached by NZFSA as a precedent. Perhaps much more importantly, however, the EFSA was faced with a horrendous problem if their conclusions favored the A1/A2 (BCM-7) hypothesis: For example, (a) it would send a panic message to the public not to consume A1 milk ... that a potential health risk was involved; (b) it would turn the dairy industry totally upside down ... telling them that they had to convert the dairy herds, literally worldwide, to A2 producers ... a process that would be incredibly expensive and would take as much as ten years to accomplish; (c) an immediate risk assessment and evaluation would be essential; (d) it would place a sudden and immediate burden on government and regulatory agencies to inspect, monitor, and regulate; (e) it would require the creation of an extensive public awareness and information program, and (f) it would require labeling of milk and milk products to identify A1 and/or A2 content, including a statement of risk assessment.

Putting all this together, yes, it was predictable that they would choose a conclusion that would diffuse all these potential problems and responsibilities ... in the hope that it would all 'blow away in the wind'.

Now, who put this report together? The eight authors are identified as the 'DATEX Working Group on β-casomorphins', and are, as listed in the report: Ivano De Noni, Richard J. FitzGerald, Hannu J.T. Kornonen, Yves Le Roux, Chris T. Livesey, Inga Thorsdottir, Daniel Tome', and Renger Witkamp. Keith Woodford, once again the relentless investigator, concludes that five could be classed as dairy scientists with strengths in bio-chemistry, two were trained in veterinary faculties and now specialize in toxicology and pharmacology, and one is a nutritionist (Inga Thorsdottir, from Iceland). One cannot help but be a little skeptical about dairy scientists working on a study that could potentially turn their industry inside-out ... and it may even be suggested that careers and job positions may be at stake. A veterinary background ... ?? ... with a specialty in toxicology and pharmacology ... ?? ... does this sound appropriate?

Interestingly, I. Thorsdottir is listed in the EFSA report's own references as the author or co-author of two studies related to the subject matter at hand, with very different conclusions from that of the report. After searching the literature, I found two additional studies authored or co-authored by Thorsdottir, again involving research in the same field. I have reviewed these studies in an earlier section in this chapter. All four studies strongly supported the A1/A2 milk (BCM-7) hypothesis.

Another author was Ivano De Noni from Italy. My own research revealed that this author had also been involved in research which supported the A1/A2 milk (BCM-7) hypothesis. He was the sole author of a study published in the journal Food Chemistry in 2008 entitled *Release of β-casomorphins 5 and 7 during simulated gastro-intestinal digestion of bovine β-casein variants and milk-based infant formulas.* His finding was that the β-casomorphins 5 and 7 were released from only the A1 and B genetic variants of milk β-casein.

However, it seems that only Thorsdittor and De Noni had been involved in any previous studies concerning the A1/A2 (BCM-7) issue. And, amazingly, both of these author's prior studies reached conclusions supportive of the A1/A2 (BCM-7) hypothesis. As Woodford points out, where are the epidemiologists, the diabetes and heart disease specialists, the neurologists, or those who are specialists in food intolerance and leaky gut syndrome?

So, you ask: "How could these two authors, having been extensively involved with research supporting the A1/A2 milk (BCM-7) hypothesis, then agree with the conclusions of the EFSA report that directly contradicts their own conclusions from previous studies?"

One startling peculiarity of the study was that nowhere could I find a recommendation or an appeal for additional studies. Considering the

209

over-all conclusion that the hypothesis is not proven, or is inconclusive, it would then make sense that additional study is desired. Via a quick run-through of the entire report I found 17 statements overtly implying that there was a need for additional research. Yet there was no appeal for further research, and the wording of the report seems to carefully avoid such an appeal. 'Recommendations' was listed in the table of contents as the very last section, and it was here that I hoped to find a recommendation for additional research. But instead, the 'Recommendation' contained only two sentences, which was a word-for-word repeat of the conclusion, (quoted above) saying nothing about the need for additional research. My own conclusion is that the 535 references were listed as a way of saying "no more study is necessary ... we already have 535 studies".

In addition, the study repeatedly stated that this or that was not *proven*, or that *cause and effect* was not established. For an exploratory study concerned primarily with risk assessment, this is very strange language. First, we know that absolute proof, especially proof of a *causal* relationship, is very elusive in scientific investigation. As I have pointed out, beginning in Chapter One, a bona-fide cause and effect relationship is almost never achieved in scientific investigation, and is not even insisted on as the primary goal. This is one reason we use statistical techniques ... to give us some sort of confidence that we are on the right track, and to give some sort of measure of our degree of success.

Secondly, one would assume that the EFSA is truly interested in *risk* as a first step ... after all, this is what they *say* is their main objective ... to assess risk ... so if potential *risk* is identified (not proof or certainty) then they should be the first to jump to attention.

There are a number of other grounds on which the report could be criticized ... but it is almost beside the point. The study and its conclusions were clearly pre-designed to placate the public and researchers by summing up the issue with 'there is no need for alarm', 'no risk assessment is warranted', and 'everyone can go on happily drinking their A1 milk without concern' ... and that the dairy industry can continue to produce it.

Sounds almost OK ... except for one small matter ... how about my and your health ?? .... how about the health of our babies and children ?? .... and future generations ?? ... and how about the increasing millions that suffer and *will* suffer from diabetes, heart disease, autism, schizophrenia, and other neurological disorders ?? Should someone be perhaps thinking about the responsibility ?? Ugh !! .... what a nasty word !!

5. **The Current Situation**

It seems that the EFSA report has put many minds at ease, and, as with NZFSA, there is no pressure to make a risk assessment or to get excited about the potential health risk of consuming A1 milk.

No call for additional research is being announced either. In fact, there has even been a recommendation that public funds should not be spent on further studies.

Fonterra, in the meantime, has been growing even larger, and expanding their marketing ever and ever wider, and becoming even more dominant as a dairy industry giant.

A2 Corporation has also been quietly increasing its footholds and trying to move into markets in other countries. They have succeeded in forming a couple of mergers with Australian companies, and have gained partial access to the Japanese market. However, their marketing attempt with Hy-Vee supermarkets in the U.S. was abandoned. And the proposal to market A2 milk in Korea under the 'Lotte' brand fell through. One apparent problem was that they could not guarantee the purity of their A2 milk ... testing milk samples and preventing contamination by A1 milk is an issue. At the present time A2 milk is being marketed only in New Zealand and Australia. A2 Corporation reported a loss of $717,172 (Australian dollars) for the first half of 2010. (A2 Corp, 2010)

Even Dr. Woodford seems to have taken a rest on the A1/A2 issue, and all is relatively quiet. No new major studies have surfaced ... the last one was the Russian Kost et al study mentioned above (2009), which showed an association between BCM-7 and a delay in psychomotor development in infants.

Concerning the situation in the dairy industry, Woodford reported the following to the International Farm Management Association at their 16th Conference, held in Ireland late 2007:

"INNOVATION FOR FUTURE PROFIT: Approximately 500 New Zealand (NZ) dairy farmers are converting their herds to eliminate production of A1 beta-casein within the milk. The alternative beta-casein is A2 beta-casein, and the associated milk is known as A2 milk. A2 milk can be considered the original milk before a mutation affected some antecedents of modern European breeds. A1 beta-casein and its derivative beta-casomorphin7 (BCM7) have been implicated in numerous health issues including Type 1 diabetes, heart disease and autism. There are now more than 100 relevant papers in peer reviewed journals. The broader NZ herd is also drifting away from A1 beta-casein production due to a serendipitous association between genetic merit as measured in NZ and A2 beta-casein. There is no evidence of this occurring in other countries. The farmer decisions can be structured using concepts of risk management and decision theory. However, analysis is complicated by uncertainty as to future premiums/discounts associated with A2/A1 milk. Outside of NZ most farmers know nothing about this issue."

Keith Woodford maintains a website entitled 'Posts from Keith Woodford' at www.keithwoodford.wordpress.com

Additional references ... with conclusions and comments ... for Chapter Four

Milk proteins associated with IDDM and autoimmune response

Fava, D.; Leslie, R.D.; Pozzilli, P.; *Relationship between dairy product consumption and incidence of IDDM in childhood in Italy,* Diabetes Care, 1994, December; 17(12): 1488-90. This is an early study by Pozzilli and his group on the relationship between dairy product consumption and the incidence of IDDM, before they had investigated the 7-amino acid peptide fragment at position 60 through 66 in A1 milk.

Glarum, M.; Robinson, B.H.; Martini, J.M.; *Could bovine serum albumin be the initiating antigen ultimately responsible for the development of insulin-dependent diabetes mellitus?* Diabetes Research, 1989, March; 10(3): 103-7. Conclusion: "Analysis of the amino-acid homology in relation to the DR/DQ allotypes found in the human population gave a strong correlation between the combined DR and DQ homology score with bovine serum albumin and the incidence of insulin-dependent diabetes mellitus."

Karges, W.; Hammond-McKibben, D.; Gaedigk, R.; Shibuya, N.; Cheung, R.; Dosch, H.M.; *Loss of self-tolerance to ICA69 in non-obese diabetic mice,* Diabetes, 1997, October; 46(10): 1548-56. This study confirms that T cell response to both pancreatic beta-cell antigens and milk proteins can demonstrate mimicry. This supports the hypothesis that an auto immune response may inadvertently attack both a milk protein peptide and the pancreatic beta-cells.

212

Karlsson, M.G.; Garcia, J.; Ludvigsson, J.; *Cows' milk proteins cause similar Th1- and Th2-like immune response in diabetic and healthy children,* Diabetologia, 2001, September; 44(9): 1140-7. This study found that the T-cell immune response to ABBOS milk protein peptide was similar for both diabetic and healthy children. Conclusion: "Thus, our results do not support the hypothesis that cows' milk antigens are important for the immune process associated with Type 1 diabetes." Another interpretation of the same data could be that the immune response was the same for children who had diabetes and *those who had not yet developed diabetes.* Once again, the ABBOS may be the wrong peptide investigated, but instead should be the BCM-7 peptide.

Karlsson, M.G.; Ludvigsson, J.; *The ABBOS-peptide from bovine serum albumin causes an IFN-gamma and IL-4 mRNA response in lymphocytes from children with recent onset of type 1 diabetes,* Diabetes Research and Clinical Practice, 2000, March; 47(3): 199-207. This is another study which supports the hypothesis that it is the ABBOS milk protein peptide that is responsible for an autoimmune attack of the pancreatic beta-cells, although ABBOS was not found to trigger a specific 'T-cell' response. Conclusion: "ABBOS may have a role as a reactive epitope in the upregulation of the autoimmune process against the beta-cells but ABBOS does not seem to cause any specific Th1 response." This would seem to suggest that the ABBOS peptide is the wrong one being investigated.

Monetini, L.; Cavallo, M.G.; Stefanini, L.; Ferrazzoli, F.; Bizzarri, C.; Marietti, G.; Curro, V.; Cervoni, M.; Pozzilli, P.; IMDIAB Group; *Bovine beta-casein antibodies in breast- and bottle-fed infants: their relevance in Type 1 diabetes,* Diabetes/Metabolism Research and Reviews, 2001, Jan-Feb; 17(1): 51-4. Antibody response to beta-casein was measured in 96 infants and children under different environmental factors. This is one of a number of studies which were led by P. Pozzilli ... in this study evidence is submitted that high levels of beta-casein antibodies are found in diabetic infants.

Padberg, S.; Schumm-Draeger, P.M.; Petzokdt, R.; Becker, F.; Federlin, K.; *The significance of A1 and A2 antibodies against beta-casein in type 1 diabetes mellitus,* Deutsche Medizinische Wochenschrigt, 1999, December 17; 124(50): 1518-21. A clinical analysis of 287 patients with IDDM, 386 siblings, 477 individual parents, and 107 healthy controls. Conclusion: "Because the A1 variant of beta-casein correlates with the onset of IDDM, but can also occur in normal controls, this may confirm the hypothesis of a defective oral immunotolerance to cow's milk antigens in IDDM." The suggestion is that the autoimmune response to beta-casein is due to a defect in the immune system, thus leading to IDDM.

Persaud, D.R.; Barranco-Mendoza, A.; *Bovine serum albumin and insulin-dependent diabetes mellitus; is cow's milk a possible toxicological causative agent of diabetes?* Food Chemistry and Toxicology, 2004, May; 42(5): 707-14. This study proposes that bovine serum albumin (BSA) in the presence of ABBOS, a peptide segment of the same protein, may be a trigger of the autoimmune attack on the pancreatic beta-cells. Conslusion: "Instead, IDDM is most likely the result of oxidative stress due to high local levels of nitric oxide and oxygen radicals on the beta-cells of the pancreas, which eventually leads to their destruction." This is a similar, yet alternative explanation compared with the BCM-7 hypothesis. Again, the ABBOS peptide may be the wrong one being investigated.

Winer, S.; Gunaratnam, L.; Astsatourov, I.; Cheung, R.K.; Kubiak, V.; Karges, W.; Hannond-McKibben, D.; Gaedigk, R. Grazian, D.; Trucco, M.; Becker, D.J.; Dosch, H.M.; *Peptide dose, MHC affinity, and target self-antigen expression are critical for effective immunotherapy of nonobese diabetic mouse prediabetes,* Journal of Immunology, 2009, October 1: 165(7): 4086-94. This study showed that therapeutic doses of the ABBOS peptide could have a protective effect on prediabetes. Once again, ABBOS may be the wrong milk peptide being investigated.

BCM-7 and neurological function and behavior

Kost, N.V.; Sokolov, O.Y.; Kurasova, O.B.; Dmitriev, A.D,; Tarakanova, J.N.; Gabaeva, M.V.; Zolotarev, Y.A.; Dadayan, A.K.; Grachev, S.A.; Korneeva, E.V.; Mikheeva, I.G.; Zozulya, A.A.; *Beta-casomorphins-7 in infants on different type of feeding and different levels of psychomotor development,* Peptides, 2009, October; 30(10): 1854-60. This study found that infants with residues of bovine irBCM (synthetic form of BCM-7) from commercial infant formulas showed delay in psychomotor development. Conclusion: "The data indicate that breast feeding has an advantage over artificial feeding for infants' development during the first year of life and support the hypothesis for deterioration of bovine casomorphin elimination as a risk factor for delay in psychomotor development and other diseases such as autism."

Zozulia, A.A.; Meshavkin, V.K.; Sokolov Olu; Kost, N.V.; *(Naloxone-induced suppression of the behavioral manifestation of serotoninergic system hperactivation by beta-casomorphin-7 in mice)*, Eksp Klin Farmakol, 2009, Mar-Apri; 72(2): 3-5. A dose of the BCM-7 peptide to mice was shown to alter standard behavior response tests (the head-twitch test) in mice, which effect was blocked by subsequent application of the opioid suppressant drug, naloxone. Conclusion: "Thus, the influence of casomorphins on the serotoninergic system in vivo has been demonstrated for the first time."

A1 and A2 milk, BCM-7, and heart disease

Taliford, K.A.; Berry, C.L.; Thomas, A.C.; Campbell, J.H.; *A casin variant in cow's milk is atherogenic*, Atherosclerosis, 2003, September; 170(1): 11-2. Sixty rabbits were divided into 10 groups and fed different concentrations of A1 and A2 beta-caseins. The rabbits fed the A1 variant beta-casein had significantly higher concentrations of arterial plaque. Conclusion: "It is concluded that beta-casein A1 is atherogenic compared with beta-casein A2."

Ven,, B.J.; Skeaff, C.M.; Brown, R.; Mann, J.I.; Green, T.J.; *A comparison of the effects of A1 and A2 beta-casein protein variants on blood cholesterol concentrations in New Zealand adults*, Atherosclerosis, 2006, September: 188(1): 175-8. A randomized cross-over trial of 55 adults over two 41/2 weeks periods. Conclusion: "We found no evidence that dairy products containing beta-casein A1 or A2 exerted differential effects on plasma cholesterol concentrations in humans."

BCM-7 and asthma, mucus formation

Bartley, J.; McGlashan, S.R.; *Does milk increase mucus production?* Medical Hypotheses, 2010, April, Vol. 74, Issue 4: 732-34 Hypothesis presentation. Conclusion: BCM-7 may be linked to increased respiratory tract mucus production and asthma.

References used in the text for Chapter Four

A2 Corporation; 2010 Mid-year Report, Available online from the A2 Corporation website

Beales, P.E.; Elliott, R.B.; Flohe', S.; Hill, J.P.; Kolb, H.; Pozzilli,P.; Wang, G.S.; Wasmuth, H.; Scott, F.W.; *A multi-centre, blinded international trial of the effect of A1 and A2 β-casein variants on diabetes incidence in two rodent models of spontaneous Type 1 diabetes,* Diabetologia, 2002, Vol. 45, No. 9, September

Berton, P.; Barnard, N.D.; Mills, M.; *Racial bias in federal nutrition policy, Part I: The public health implications of variations in lactase persistence,* Journal of the National Medical Association, 1999, March; 91(3): 151-7.

Birgisdottir, B.E.; Hill, J.P.; Thorsson, A.V.; Thorsdottir, I.; *Lower consumption of cow milk protein A1 beta-casein at 2 years of age, rather than consumption among 11- to 14-year old adolescents, may explain the lower incidence of type 1 diabetes in Iceland than in Scandinavia,* Annals of Nutrition and Metabolism, 2008; 50(3): 177-83

Birgisdottir, B.E.; Hill, J.P.; Thorsdottir, I.; *Variations in consumption of cow milk proteins and lower incidence of Type 1 diabetes in Iceland vs the other 4 Nordic countries,* Diabetes, Nutrition & Metabolism - Clinical & Experimental, 2002, August; 15(4): 240-5

Cade, R.; Privette, M.; Fregly, M.; Rowland, N.; Sun, Z.; Zele, V.; Wagemaker, H.; Edelstein, C.; *Autism and schizophrenia: intestinal disorders,* Nutritional Neuroscience, 2000; 3:57-72

Cavallo, M.G.; Fava, D.; Monetini, L.; Pozzilli, P.; *Cell-mediated immune response to beta casein in recent-onset insulin-dependent diabetes: implications for disease pathogenesis,* Lancet, 1996, October 5; 348(9032): 926-8. This was a clinical study of 47 patients with recent-onset IDDM and 36 healthy controls. Interpretation: "The association between IDDM and early consumption of cow's milk may be explaine by the generation of a specific immune response to beta casein. Exposure to cows' milk triggers a cellular and humoral anti-beta casein immune response which may cross-react with a beta-cell antigen. It is of interest that sequence homologies exist between beta casein and several beta-cell molecules."

Dr. Paolo Pozzilli is Professor of Diabetes and Clinical Research at the Centre for Diabetes at Barts and The London School of Medicine & Dentistry, London , and Professor of Endocrinology & Metabolic Diseases at the University Campus Bio-Medico in Rome , Italy.

He is the Delegate for University Campus Bio-Medico, Permanent Conference of Rectors of the Italian Universities (CRUI), Member Scientific Advisory Board, Graduate School in Molecular Medicine,

University of Ulm and Member Advisory Board, International Diabetes Federation, Group for Diabetes in the Youth. He coordinates the International PhD programme in Endocrinology and Metabolic Diseases between Queen Mary University of London, University Campus Bio-Medico in Rome and the University of Ulm, Germany.

Dr. Pozzilli is also the European Editor of Diabetes Metabolism Research & Reviews and Associate Editor of Nutrition Metabolism and Cardiovascular Disease. He is the Review Editor for the International Diabetes Monitor and Member of the International Commission of the Italian Society of Endocrinology.

He was the recipient of several awards amongst which the Andrew Cudworth Memorial Prize of the British Diabetic Association (1986), the G.B. Morgagni Prize, Young Investigator Award of the European Association of Metabolism (1989), the SID Prize 1994 (Italian Society of Diabetes), the Karol Marcinkowski Medal of the "Poznan Academy of Medicine"(1997), the Mary Jane Kugel Award, Juvenile Diabetes Research Foundation, USA (2003 and 2006) and the Diabetes Honoris Causa, Paulescu Foundation & Romanian Society of Diabetes (2007).

Dr Pozzilli is involved with a wide assortment of studies in the field of diabetes, including animal studies and the use of stem cell therapy.

Dalziel, Honorable Lianne; Report to the New Zealand Office of the Minister for Food Safety, April 4th, 2008

De Noni, I.; *Release of β-casomorphins 5 and 7 during simulated gastro-intestinal digestion of bovine β-casein variants and milk-based infant formula.* Food Chemistry, 2008, October 15; Vol. 110, Issue 4: 897-903

Dubynin, V.A.; Malinovskala, I.V.; Beliaeva, IuA.; Stovolosov, I.S.; Bespalova, ZhD.; Andreeva, L.A.; Kamenskil, A.A.; Miasoedov, N.F.; *Delayed effect of exorphins on learning of albino rat pups,* Izv Akad Nauk Ser Biol, 2008, Jan-Feb; (1): 53-60

Elliott, R.B.; *Diabetes – A man made disease,* Medical Hypotheses, 2006, Vol. 67, Issue 2: 388-91

Elliott, R.B.; Harris, D.P.; Hill, J.P.; Bibby, N.J.; Wasmuth, H.E.; *Type 1 (insulin-dependent) diabetes mellitus and cow milk: casein variant consumption,* Diabetologia, 1999, March; 42(3): 292-6. This was the preliminary study to the Laugesen and Elliott study of 2003.

Elliott, R.B.; Laugesen, M.; *The influence of consumption of A1 β-casein on heart disease and Type 1 diabetes – the authors reply*, The New Zealand Medical Journal, 2003, March; Vol. 116, No. 1179

Elliott, R.B.; Martin, J.M.; *Dietary protein: a trigger of insulin-dependent diabetes in the BB rat?* Diabetologia, 1984; 26: 297-99.

European Food Safety Authority (EFSA); *Review of the potential health impact of β-casomorphins and related peptides,* Report of the DATEX Working Group on β-casomorphins, January 29th, 2009. Available online via the EFSA website.

Formaggioni, A.; Summer, A.; Malacarne, M.; Mariani, P.; *Milk Protein Polymorphism: Detection and Diffusion of the Genetic Variants in Bos Genus,* Instituto di Zootecnica, Alimentazione e Nutrizione, Universita degli Studi, 1999.
www.unipr.it/arpa/facvet/annali/1999/formaggioni/formaggioni.htm

Ng-Kwai-Hang, K.F.; Grosclaude, F.; *Genetic polymorphism of milk proteins,* Chapter 16 in Advanced Dairy Chemistry: Volume 1: Proteins, Parts A & B., Fox, P.F.; McSweeney, P.; Editors, 2003 (3rd ed.)

Henschen, A.; Lottspeich, F.; Branti, V.; Teschemacher, H.; *Novel opioid peptides derived from casein (beta-casomorphins), II. Structure of active components from bovine casein peptone,* Hoppe-Seyler's Zeitschrift fur physiologische Chemie, 1979, September; 360(9): 1217-24.

Howard, A.A.; Hoover, D.R.; Anastos, K.; Wu, X.; Shi, Q.; Strickler, H.D.; Cole, S.R.; Cohen, M.H.; Kovacs, A.; Augenbraun, M.; Latham, P.S.; Tien, P.C.; *The effects of opiate use and hepatitis C virus infection on risk of diabetes mellitus in the women's interagency HIV study.,* Journal of Acquired Immune Deficiency Syndromes, 2010, June; 54(2): 152-9

Iwan, M.; Jarmolowska, B.; Bielikowicz, K.; Kostyra, E.; Kostyra, H.; Kaczmarski, M.; *Transport of micro-opioid receptor agonists and antagonis peptides across Caco-2 monolayer,* Peptides, 2008, June; 29(6); 1042-7.

Karjaleinen, J.; Martin, J.M.; Knip, M.; Ilonen, J.; Robinson, B.H.; Savilahtl, E.; Akerblom, H.K.; Dosch, H.M.; *A bovine albumin peptide as a possible trigger of insulin-dependent diabetes mellitus.* New England Journal of Medicine, 1992, July 30; 327(5): 302-7

Kiddy, C.A.; Peterson, R.F.; Kopfler, F.C.; *Genetic control of the variants of β-casein A,* Journal of Dairy Science, 49, 742, 1966

Kost, N.V.; Sokolov, O.Y. Kurasova, O.B.; Dimitriev, A.D.; Tarakanova, J.N.; Gabaeva, M.V.; Zolotarev, Y.A.; Dadayan, A.K.; Grachev, S.A.; Korneeva, E.V.; Mikheeva, I.F.; Zozulya, A.A.; *Beta-casomorphins-7 in infants on different type of feeding and different levels of psychomotor development.* Peptides, 2009, October; 30(10): 1854-60

Laugesen, M.; Elliot, R.; *Ischaemic heart disease, Type 1 diabetes, and cow milk A1 beta-casein,* New Zealand Medical Journal, 2003, January 24; 116(1168): U295. This is the study that finally drew attention to the A1, A2 milk variant and the BCM-7 molecule issue.

McLachlan, C.N.; *Beta-casein A1, ischaemich heart disease mortality, and other illnesses,* Medical Hypotheses, 2001, February; 56(2): 262-72

McLachlan, C.N.; Olson, F.; *Setting the record straight: A1 β-casein, heart disease and diabetes,* The New Zealand Medical Journal, 2003, March, Vol. 116, No. 1170

Meisel, H.; FitzGerald, R.J.; *Opioid peptides encrypted in intact milk protein sequences,* British Journal of Nutrition, 2000; 84, Suppl. 1, S27-S31.

New Zealand Food Safety Authority (NZFSA); *Beta casein A1 and A2 in milk and human health: Lay Summary,* Lay Summary to the Swinburn Report, Available online at www.nfsa.govt.nz/policy-law/projects/a1-a2milk/lay-summary.htm

Ng-Kwai-Hang, K.F.; Hayes, J.F.; Moxley, J.E.; Monardes, H.G.; *Association of genetic variants of casein and milk serum proteins with milk, fat, and protein production by dairy cattle,* Journal of Dairy Science, 1984, April; 67(4): 835-40.

Ng-Kwai-Hang, K.F.; Grosclaude, F.; *Genetic polymorphism of milk proteins,* Chapter 16 of *Advance Dairy Chemistry,* pp 737-814, Fox, P.F. and McSweeney, P.L.H.; editors; published by Kluwer Academic/Plenum Publishers, New York, 2002

Noel, R.J. Jr; Rivera-Amill, V.; Buch, S.; Kumar, A.; *Opiates, immune system, acquired immunodeficiency syndrome, and nonhuman primate model,* Journal of Neurovirol, 2008, August; 14(4): 279-85.

Peterson, R.F; Kopfler, F.C.; *Detection of new types of β-casein by polyacrylamide gel electrophoresis at acid pH: a proposed nomenclature,* Biochemical and Biophysical Research Communications, 22, 388-392, 1966

Scott, F.; Kolb, H.; *A1 β-casein milk and Type 1 diabetes: causal relationship probed in animal models,* New Zealand Medical Journal, 2003, March; Vol. 116, No. 1170

Shattock, P.; Kennedy, A.; Rowell, F.; Berney, T.; *Role of neuropeptides in autism and their relationships with classical transmitters,* Brain Dysfunction, 1990, 3:328-46

Sidor, K.; Jarmolowska, B.; Kaczmarski, M.; Kostyra, E.; Iwan, M.; Kostyra, H.; *Content of beta-casomorphins in milk of women with a history of allergy,* Pediatric Allergy and Immunology, 2008, November; 19(7): 587-91.

Sienkiewicz-Szlapka, S.; Jarmolowska, B.; Krawczuk, H.; Bielkowicz, K.; *Transport of bovine milk-derived opioid peptides across a Caco-2 monolayer,* International Dairy Journal, 2009, April; Vol. 19, Issue 4: 252-57

Steinerova, A.; Stozik, F.; Racek, J.; Tatzbar, F.; Zima, T.; Stetina, R.; *Antibodies against Oxidized LDL in infants.* Clinical Chemistry, 2001; 47: 1137-8

Sun, Z.; Cade, J.R.; Fregly, M.J.; Privette, R.M.; *Beta-casomorphin induces Fos-like immunoreactivity in discrete brain regions relevant to schizophrenia and autism,* Autism, 1999, 3(1): 67-81

Swinburn, B.; *Beta casein A1 and A2 in milk and human health, Report to New Zealand Food Safety Authority,* July 13th, 2004. Available online from the NZFSA website.

Taliford, K.A.; Berry, C.L.; Thomas, A.C.; Campbell, J.H.; *A casein variant in cow's milk is atheogenic.* Atherosclerosis, 2003, September; 170(1): 13-9

Thompson, M.P.; Kiddy, C.A.; Johnston, J.O.; Weinberg, R.M.; *Genetic polymorphism in caseins of cow's milk. II. Confirmation of the genetic control of beta-casein variations,* Journal of Dairy Science; 47: 378-81, 1964.

Thorsdottir, I.; Birgisdottir, B.E.; Johannsdottir, I.M.; Harris, D.P.; Hill, J.; Steingrimsdottir, L.; Thorsson, A.V.; *Different β-caseub fractions in Icelandic versus Scandinavian cow's milk may influence diabetogenicity of cow's milk in infancy and explain low incidence of insulin-dependent diabetes mellitus in Iceland.* Pediatrics, 2000, 106(4): 719-24

Thorsdottir, I.; Reykdal, O.; *Food and the low incidence of IDDM in Iceland*, Scandivanvian Journal of Nutrition/Naringsforskning, 1997, 4: 97

Torreilles, J.; Guerin, M.C.; *Casein-derived peptides can promote human LDL oxidation by a peroxidase-dependent and metal-independent process.* Comptes Rendus des Seances de la Societe de Biologie et des ses Filiales (Paris), 1995; 189(5): 933-42

Truswell, A.S.; *The A2 milk case: a critical review,* European Journal of Clinical Nutrition, 2005; 59, 623-31

Truswell, A.S.; *Reply: The A2 milk case: a critical review,* European Journal of Clinical Nutrition, 2006; 60, 924-25

Van Eenenw, A.; Fernando-Medrano, J.; *Milk Protein Polymorphisms in California Dairy Cattle,* Journal of Dairy Sciences, Vol. 74, No. 5, 1991

Wang, J.; Barke, R.A.; Ma, J.; Charboneau, R.; Roy, S.; *Opiate abuse, innate immunity, and bacterial infectious diseases,* Archivum Immunologiae Et Tharapiae Experimentalis, 2008, Sept-Oct; 56(5): 299-309.

Woodford, K.; *An invited plenary paper to the International Diabetes Federation Western Pacific Congress, Wellington, 2 April, 2008.*

Woodford, K.B.; *A critique of Truswell's A2 milk review,* European Journal of Clinical Nutrition; 60(3): 437-39

Woodford, K.; *A2 Milk, Farmer Decisions, and Risk Management; Innovation For Future Profit;* A paper presented at the 16th Conference of the International Farm Management Association, held in Ireland, 2007

Summary Statement for Chapter Four, the 'Ugly'

The compelling new evidence and studies leading to and supporting the A1/A2 millk (BCM-7) hypothesis constitutes a whole new dimension to the question of whether or not we should drink milk. 'All the evidence is *not* in' ... of course ... we urgently need more research and more well-designed studies. But there is enough study and evidence already accumulated to warrant careful consideration ... and caution.

What future science reveals will be of great interest and importance.

CHAPTER FIVE

CONCLUSIONS, IMPLICATIONS, AND CALL FOR ACTION

.... What is at stake is your and my health ... and the health of our babies, and our children ... and of generations to come. And what about the increasing millions who suffer and will suffer from diabetes, heart disease, and neurological disorders.

.... It may not be so much a question of what science will eventually conclude ... although this is extremely important ... but may be more a matter of consumers knowing the truth, being protected, and having a choice.

Imperfect foods ... insights from nutritional anthropolgy

Learning about the foods we eat is a fascinating study, full of contradictions, curiosities, and startling insights. Some of our most favorite foods, if not prepared correctly or consumed in too large a quantity, can be downright dangerous. And it seems that no single food gives us a total of everything we need ... there is really no such thing as a 'perfect food'.

One of my favorite examples of this apparent paradox is the wonderful soybean. It is truly a nutritious plant. Yet, the raw soybean contains a strong 'trypsin inhibitor', which prevents the enzyme trypsin from performing its role in breaking down ingested protein into its component amino acids in the small intestine. It will not only prevent the protein in the soybean from being digested, but potentially the protein in the rest of the food mass that is eaten at the same time, if the soybean content is large enough. Historically, of course, no one ever knew about this in a scientific sense, but populations that consumed the soybean knew by trial and error and traditional use that the soybean was not to be eaten raw. And thus the Japanese, for example, cook or roast the soybean, or make other products such as tofu … which neutralizes the tripsin inhibitor and makes the soybean safe to eat. If the soybean was to be eaten raw, and in large enough quantities for a long enough time, it would kill us!

When the allied forces were recruiting soldiers in Pakistan during WWII they encountered a large number of young recruits that looked like pre-teen boys, baby-faced and unnaturally short in stature. Investigation by medical teams revealed that these men were severely deficient in the mineral zinc, and further study showed that most of the Pakistani population were similarly lacking in zinc. The answer to the puzzle "why?" was discovered to be linked with a food that had been recently introduced and much consumed … corn. Our common raw corn kernel contains a strong negatively charged phytate structure that binds the positively charged bi-valent zinc, and prevents its absorption into the body … it is instead excreted along with the corn fiber as fecal matter. The Pakistanis had imported corn as a new food, but had failed to import the technique of how to neutralize the binding effect of raw corn fibers. The indigenous peoples of South and Central American, from where corn had originated, treated the corn and corn flour with lime … it was a traditional, long practiced technique. They didn't really know why they did it, but it was what their mothers had done, and the mothers before … it was a cultural tradition. We can now explain why the lime neutralizes the zinc-binding property of corn more scientifically: the lime has a very high ph (is alkaline) and by raising the ph of the corn the negative charge of the corn fiber molecule is weakened and no longer binds the zinc. The Mexicans, for example, treat the corn and their tortillas with lime, which is also the reason why tortillas have a higher calcium content than the corn it is made from … lime is mostly calcium carbonate.

I have heard many folks, particularly vegetarians, extol the nutrient advantages of the remarkable almond nut. I smile when I hear this, because the nut of the almond tree has an especially interesting history. And it is not as nearly the 'almost perfect food' that some think it is. For example, it has absolutely no vitamin C, D, A, nor K, it has a higher percentage of saturated fat that whole milk (3.7%), no omega-3 and very little omega-6, and its protein is lacking in the amino acid methionine and possibly limiting in lysine and cystine as well (compared with egg protein). But even more fascinating, the ancestor to the modern-day almond was in fact a deadly poison … it could not be consumed by humans at all. Now, somewhere along the line, historically, a mutation in the almond tree rendered its nut safe to eat, and this beneficial mutation (beneficial to us, but not the almond tree) was successfully nurtured by early agriculturists to become the dominant variant. However, prior to that event, eating the nut of the almond tree would surely send one to their maker.

There are many other similar stories to tell, but the message is that the foods we cherish and consider so valuable can often have negative quirks as well. And so it is with the case of cow's milk. Again borrowing from Melanie DuPuis, the story of milk is *not* a 'perfect story'. Nor should it be a 'downfall story'. The controversy surrounding milk and dairy products will not be easily resolved, perhaps not resolved at all ... there are a large number of valid pros and cons, and our scientific understanding still has sizable gaps.

Comparing the literature ... the pros and cons

In Chapter Two, the 'Good', I tried to present a fair appraisal of that side of the debate, and the supportive studies are indeed impressive. The studies and arguments which cast doubt on the proverbial good of milk are also impressive, which I have presented in Chapter Three, the 'Bad'. In all fairness, the number of studies and the strength of the conclusions tend to favor the 'good'. So how do we reach our own conclusion, and which side of the debate should we favor ?

I personally feel that the discovery of the differences in casein variants and the BCM-7 peptide, however, presents a whole new factor. I cannot help think that if the many studies noted in chapter two *and* three were done again, with awareness of the new knowledge about and supporting the A1/A2 milk (BCM-7) hypothesis, their study designs, the questions asked, and the conclusions arrived at ... all might have turned out very different. I also cannot help but consider that the pro arguments and studies are all under the influence of the 'grand paradigm' ... the paradigm, or conventional wisdom, in which 'milk' is held is such great esteem, and it's 'goodness' unquestionable.

But, as I suggest above, perhaps it is not important to arrive at a definitive 'yes' or 'no' to the question of whether we should, or should not, drink milk. We can choose a softer, middle-of-the-road approach ... and base our ultimate personal opinion on the 'imperfect story'.

Conclusions

The conclusions in this chapter are mine. You, the reader, may have formed a very different opinion, and that is of course your prerogative ...

it is the way it should be. What is important is that we have entered a discussion, a dialogue, and I have presented the information and the pros and cons as best I could.

The controversy surrounding the production and consumption of cow's milk and dairy products can be divided into fourteen major issues, which have been identified and debated in the previous chapters. The following is a summary and brief concluding discussion of each:

1. Is cow's milk a traditional human food, and are our physiologies genuinely adapted to its consumption?

There is no question that the domestication of the *Bos Taurus* and the consumption of the milk from its' udder is a recent event in an evolutionary perspective. And yes, lactose intolerance, cow's milk allergy, and other problems that some people have with the digestion and utilization of milk are strong indicators that our physiologies are not designed for consuming cow's milk, especially into adulthood. However, there is good evidence that at least some populations of humans have acquired the necessary genetic alteration to accommodate the digestion of bovine milk, and most humans even without the genetic modification (can produce lactase into adulthood) are able to tolerate modest amounts. It seems we do have the ability to adapt.

2. Is cow's milk really 'nature's most perfect food'?

Heaven's no !! As outlined in Chapter Three, cow's milk is deficient in a number of vitamins and minerals, possibly has too much saturated fat (at least whole milk), does not provide nearly enough omega-3, or even omega-6, and its protein is limiting in methionine, cystine, tryptophan and possibly lysine. It is truly a great source for calcium, however, and that is important. Its' whey protein may also be an especially valuable protein … we are still finding out more about the advantages of whey.

3. Is cow's milk suitable for human infants?

No. And this is an emphatic no. The lesson has been long learned, and the consensus is well established … human milk is best for human babies. Formula based on cow's milk is also not recommended.

4. Does drinking milk and eating dairy products truly give us the best source of calcium, and is this calcium beneficial and/or necessary to prevent osteoporosis

Cow's milk is definitely an excellent source of needed calcium, and there are special attributes in milk that facilitate its' absorption. However, the calcium carbonate form of calcium in milk may not be the *best* absorbed, and there are other good sources for calcium. The relation of calcium to osteoporosis is still not completely understood. The more we learn about osteoporosis the more we find that it is a multi-factoral condition, and many more nutrients are specifically important to bone development and maintenance than just calcium.

5. If we are genuinely lactose intolerant, should we avoid dairy products?

Absolutely !! If one is genuinely lactose intolerant and suffers from the consumption of cow's milk and milk products, then they should not consume this food, and especially not force it upon themselves.

6. Should the recommendation to consume dairy products also apply to those are lactose intolerant, and is it politically correct, considering that most non-white ethnic groups are lactose intolerant?

It is a mistake and is pure ethnocentrism to insist that non-white groups who are commonly lactose intolerant consume cow's milk and milk products. It is also a mistake to design food guidelines and recommendations that do not take this factor into consideration.

7. Should we follow the advice of vegetarians and not consume milk products because they are derived from animals and are not plant-based?

As I have stated, it is my own personal opinion that vegetarianism is a worthwhile goal ... it is the ideal. However, given the condition of our present-day food supply and food consumption habits, it is extremely difficult to obtain adequate amounts of all our needed nutrients by consuming plant-based foods only. A vegetarian diet places an individual at high risk for several nutrient deficiencies. It must be noted that there is no plant source for vitamin B-12. Iron and complete protein are two other nutrients in short supply in plant foods. And while calcium can be sourced from a variety of plant foods, its bioavailability is a limiting factor. My own recommendation is that a person pursuing a vegetarian diet should regularly take an all-around vitamin-mineral supplement, with extra calcium and omega-3.

8. Should we deny animal-based foods on the basis of animal rights sentiments?

I personally feel that there is something basically wrong with our practice of raising and then slaughtering animals purely to provide foods for our stomachs. I would think that we humans should by now have figured out a way to do without the need for animal meat, and especially the need to carry out the process of obtaining it under such inhumane and gross circumstances.

9. Should we decide not to purchase milk products produced and/or processed by mega-dairies or large processing companies that we feel are unscrupulous, overly profit-orientated, and produce questionable products, with questionable ingredients?

This is a tough one !! Big business can be more efficient, and make our food choices available to us at lower cost and with less contamination. On the other hand, big business can be highly manipulative and insulated from consumer concerns, and thus make the foods more expensive and with impurities that are hidden from the consumer.

10. Should we avoid cow's milk and milk products from cows treated with recombinant bovine growth hormone (rBGH), anti-biotics, and other substances.?

A major point of this entire book is that the consumer must be protected and informed. We have the right to know what is in our food, and we must be given the choices. We have the right to know if the milk or milk products we purchase and consume come from dairy cows that have been treated with rBGH or anti-biotics or other substance. If a product is from treated cows, labeling should reflect this.

11. Should we refuse to drink milk because of possible contamination with blood, pus, and manure?

I answer this one with a touch of humor. I once read that Americans eat an average about 3 pounds of insects every year ... insects that in one way or another get into our foods, which is particularly a problem with processed foods. A small amount of contamination is inevitable. The dairy industry is highly regulated and monitored, and the minimization of contamination is emphasized. A little bit of dirt, manure, straw or feed, and a touch of pus will not hurt us. On the other hand, I feel that the maximum allowed somatic cell count (SCC) level of 750,000 is too high. The U.S. standard should be more in line with that of the EU, at 400,000 per ml.

12. Should we choose not to consume milk products because current labeling (particularly in the U.S.) may not tell us the truth about what is in the product or from what cows it came from?

Yes ... the label on the product is the only way that a consumer can learn about what is in, or is not in, food products. We have a right to know, and the labels should fulfill that prerogative.

13. Are there credible links between drinking milk and eating dairy products with certain disease conditions in humans?

This gets us to Chapter Four, and the A1/A2 milk (BCM-7) hypothesis. This of course is highly controversial and the evidence is a long ways from being complete. But the risks have been identified, and there is enough evidence to warrant concern.

14. Should we avoid drinking A1 cow's milk?

Given that the risks have been identified and a good amount of evidence put together, it is surely prudent to avoid A1 cow's milk. Especially in respect to our babies and young children. The availability of the alternative A2 variant is important, and providing the availability and the choice should be a matter of utmost importance for the dairy industry, for government, and for the scientific community.

The evidence that the BCM7 peptide is the "ugly" component in A1 cow's milk and is directly linked to the chronic diseases of diabetes, heart disease, and a host of other illnesses, is becoming increasingly difficult to refute. It has reached the point where the public, health care professionals and the government cannot ignore it. It has become even more important for our dairy industry to take the initiative and to boldly confront this issue, and all its ramifications.

14. **Should we avoid dairy products because the industry leaders have been unscrupulous and have misled the consumer public and concealed data and the truth about their products, and are continuing to do so?**

We are the consumers. In a democratic society we, the people, are the most important entities. In commerce, our purchase is our vote. Yes, if the industry and commercial powers to be are not being transparent and honest, then yes, we should exercise our vote and refuse to purchase their product.

Milk .... to drink, or not to drink .... that is the question !!??

And now it is time to answer the grand question, and the title of this book: "Milk .... to drink, or not to drink ?"

When you put it all together ... the 'good', the 'bad', and the 'ugly'... it is not an easy question to answer ... especially in a 'grande finale' sense.

Personally, I feel very much the same as Woodford, Swinburn, Elliott and McLachlan ... there is simply too much good science over a very long of time to treat the issue of milk, and especially the A1/A2 milk (BCM-7) hypothesis, lightly ... or passively. And it has not only been the science directly supporting the central hypothesis ... it has been the long, steady progress of putting the pieces of the puzzle together ... a process demonstrating continuity and a progression to form a big picture.

What is clear, I feel, is that some changes are due. Cow's milk , even in the best scenario, is *not* a 'perfect food' In my estimation it doesn't even come close. But it has been one of America's favorite foods ... for a very long time. It is as American as apple pie. It is dear to the people of Europe, and other Western countries as well. And to say bad things about it hits home to our very hearts, and stirs emotion. And milk is an ingrained part of the conventional wisdom, the grand paradigm that so prevails our thinking, especially in public health policy and education, and the science that supports that policy.

The changes that need to be made are, first, to improve the quality and purity of milk products, and second, to insist on the A2 variant. There is currently a strong and growing consumer preference for 'raw' and 'organic' milk ... milk that is free of such chemicals as rBGH, anti-biotics, and pesticides. This needs to be taken more seriously by the dairy industry and government. The A1/A2 issue will not go away ... the dairy industry, again, must make changes, and our governments must promote and support the needed change.

With improvements and changes, milk may then warrant its' position as a favorite food, and be suitable to drink. Personally, I would not drink milk that I know is contaminated with rBGH and anti-biotics, nor would I drink milk that contains even a small percentage of the type A1 variant beta-casein. And I would tell my children to follow my example, and I would tell them not to drink too much, if at all ... one glass a day plus a small amount of cheese or yogurt, but never the 3, 4, and more glasses now recommended by the dairy industry and public health policy makers.

Implications

If we conclude that the drinking of cow's milk is indeed unhealthy and undesirable, then the implications are enormous.

Affect on human health

The most important implication is the effect on human health, and the individual's decision on whether or not to consume milk and/or milk products. Drinking a glass of milk, or several glasses, or soaking your bowl of cornflakes in milk, or adding it to your hot cereal, or even topping off your cup of coffee ... these eating habits have become an entrenched and favored part of American and European eating habits ... indeed, throughout a major part of the world. To suddenly discourage the intake of milk is to suggest a major shift in our eating habits.

Effect on the dairy industry

If the reader has followed through with the discussion in the previous chapters, and in this chapter, the implications for the dairy industry, government, and the scientific community are clear ... and are enormous.

Keith Woodford estimates that it would take ten years to convert a nation's dairy herds to A2 producers, given overt and focused attention. So what does the industry do in the meantime? What is to be done with all the A1 milk that will be produced in the interim? Perhaps a good percentage of the populations won't care about the possible health hazard ... or wouldn't believe that there is a risk ... and would continue to consume A1 milk. Milk products which don't have the BCM-7 casomorphin could be available as options. With some dedicated science, we may even be able to come up with ways to eliminate or neutralize the BCM-7 devil in the type A1 variant.

Or, we might simply drink a lot less milk. When the switch away from cow's milk to breastfeeding and using alternative products such as soybean or other animal milk occurred in the 1970s and 80s, the dairy industry managed to not only survive, but continued to flourish. And keep in mind that drinking fluid cow's milk in large quantities did not take place until the late 1800s, and with pasteurization in the 1920s.

A new challenge and responsibility for government, the scientific community, and educators

Governments and their regulatory agencies are faced with the task of regulating, monitoring, and promoting new research. Labeling requirements are a natural outcome. Funding for new studies must be generated and allocated.

The scientific community must also face up to the challenge, to both continue research to continue the debate and seek the truth, and to find ways to facilitate the changes more easily.

And our nations educators, at all levels, must take on the responsibility to be informed ... to be educated themselves ... and to be the bridge between the consumer and government, and with the scientific community.

A new challenge and responsibility for consumers

Yes ... we, the consumers, also face a new challenge and responsibility. We consumers need to be vocal, and to exercise our vote both politically and in the form of what we choose to purchase ... to demand change. The consumer is faced with a new responsibility ... yes, *responsibility* ... responsibility to prompt the dairy industry, the governments, *and* science in the right direction. Without push from the consumer, it may truly all 'blow away with the wind' ... which is surely what the dairy industry and government would like to see happen

Call for action

If the consumption of cow's milk is not good for us, or embodies health risks, then it is clear that we have been deceived

What is at stake is my and your health ... and the health of our babies and children ... and that of future generations. This is to say nothing of the suffering by the increasing millions of those who have or will have diabetes, heart disease, autism, schizophrenia, and other neurological disorders.

The most urgent step is to immediately spread awareness of the potential danger of the BDM-7 opiate, and of consuming A1 milk. Considering the 'head-in-the-sand' posture of agencies like the EFSA and expected resistance from the dairy industry, this is going to require pressure from the consumer public ... from you and I.

We consumers must embrace this new responsibility ... we must speak up and be heard, and place our votes appropriately ... both in the political arena and in the supermarket.

A bold new perspective

From the point of view of 'the big picture' of just where our human race is at, and our food supply, one could say that we are on the verge of entering a new era ... or at least we have the capacity and opportunity to step up to a new era. The stage has been set: the power of the consumer is greater than ever, and the responsibility of government and science, and industry, to serve the needs of the consuming public is well established. This was not always so. But thanks to the past efforts of giants like Ralph Nader, we have the framework in place. Writers such as John Robbins have promoted the awareness that something is very wrong with the way humankind organizes and implements the provision of our food supply, and even the nature of our food supply. I personally do not agree with much of his point of view and his style of research and writing, but he and others have promoted a basic public awareness.

We have the capability and the awareness to now move on, and to enter a new era, and to embrace a *bold new perspective*. This new era will characterize a strong shift away from a dependence on an animal-based diet to a more vegetarian diet, away from domination and manipulation by big business, and away from government that prefers to keep 'it's head in the sand'. There will be a new awareness about our food choices, and a concern and effort to improve the quality and nutrient density of those food choices. The new era will place the consuming public first, with a strong emphasis on consumer protection, consumer education and awareness, and a stress on consumer choice. Our educators will more actively engage in the quest for new knowledge, and will be the bridge between the consumer and government, and the scientific community. Hopefully, a new rationality will also emerge, directed at more intelligent food choices and more sensible eating habits.

References for Chapter Five

Johnson, F.E.; *Nutritional Anthropology*, Alan R. Liss, Ince, 1987

APPENDIX

About the Paradigm

The notion that scientific inquiry can be subject to bias and misinformation by the influence of strongly held points of view, doctrines, and/or beliefs by the researchers and the scientific community is a surprise to most people not familiar with scientific study, and also to many of those who *are* involved, even the scientists themselves. This was especially true in earlier times, when science and medicine were held in great esteem and their territory thought to be hallowed. This reverence suffered a great challenge when it became clear that science was subject to major shifts in direction, and that sacred tenets held to be absolute by one generation crumbled when viewed by another.

The nature of scientific progress

Probably the foremost thinker in this new way of viewing the progress of science was Thomas S. Kuhn, author of *The Copernican Revolution* (1957, 1985) and *The Structure of Scientific Revolutions* (1962, 1970, 1996). His central observation was that the progress of science jumped in revolutionary steps, in almost a generation to generation fashion, with an earlier generation of scientists dogmatically pursuing one singular pathway, or paradigm, unswayed until a newly arrived generation challenged that pathway and was able to move on to a new perspective, a new paradigm.

Thomas Kuhns' insights have become generally known and appreciated among academics, yet his observation still holds. In more recent times it has been suggested that we no longer jump from one paradigm to a totally new one, but instead we experience a *paradigm shift*. Whether it is a shift or a jump to a whole new paradigm is a matter of debate.

Nowhere is the existence of a paradigm more clear than in modern medicine, and nutrition, as taught and practiced in Europe, the United States, and other Western countries.

So .... how can this paradigm be described ... and what is wrong with it ... and how should it be changed ... or *shifted* ??

What do doctors know about nutrition ??

One characteristic of the prevailing paradigm in medical science is the reluctance to take the subject of nutrition seriously. When you or I think about bodily health, we quickly include nutrition as a key factor ... it is common sense ... yet your practicing medical doctor is not nearly so agreeable to do the same. Yes, he will eagerly discuss nutrition ... from the perspective of diet ... but *not* as a bona-fide part of medicine itself. Yes, he will recognize the disease conditions caused by outright deficiencies of essential nutrients, but more of a concession rather than an acceptance ... and he will stubbornly refuse to consider possible health benefits of additional nutrient intake beyond that needed to prevent the deficiency diseases, such as scurvy, caused by a deficiency of vitamin C, or rickets caused by very low intakes of calcium.

This failure to include nutrition as an integral part of the core of medical science can be illustrated by the dismal attempt to teach nutrition to pre-med and medical school students. As an example, the University of Hawaii is a standard, fully accredited American university, with the attached John Burns School of Medicine, and the usual undergraduate curriculums in pre-med, nursing, medical technology ... and nutrition and food science as well ... the FSHN Department where I earned my Bachelor's of Science degree in human nutrition. My nutrition curriculum was essentially the same as the pre-med curriculum, with the same courses in biology and zoology and physiology, general chemistry and organic chemistry, and biochemistry. Except that I was required to study more biochemistry and a host of specific nutrition classes. Much of my class time was therefore with pre-med students, and in study-group and study-hall sessions as well. The pre-med students were my classmates. I admired them greatly, for they were the smartest of the smart, dedicated to their studies, and intensely focused. Whenever I entered a new class at the beginning of a semester, and saw that many in the class were pre-meds, I groaned, knowing that getting an "A" is this class was going to be tough.

I noticed even from the beginning courses that the pre-med students had little interest in nutrition, per se. Yes, they would diligently study in the areas that 'brushed' alongside nutrition ... in physiology, biology, and biochemistry, but they did not delve deeper, and they were diffident to entering discussions with me about the subject of nutrition. Perhaps they were so focused on their immediate studies that they had no time to explore what was considered a non-essential subject ... or perhaps they were already attuned to omitting nutrition as a bona-fide part of medicine.

No nutrition courses were required by the pre-meds at UH, although the nursing students were obligated to take one course in their final semester. I audited that course, and knew it well, and was surprised to observe that the nursing students were reluctant to study nutrition as well. Why, I wondered at the time.

The pre-med and medical school curriculums are standardized and follow accreditation guidelines, but they are not *required* to teach nutrition. Neither does the American Medical Association require nutrition education, and knowledge of nutrition is *not* required to get through medical internship and finally become a practicing medical doctor.

Searching for some statistics about nutritional education in medical schools, I came across a study by Frank M. Torti, et al, which reported the results of a survey taken July 1999 to May 2000 of 122 U.S. medical and osteopathic medical schools (which is just about all of them ... I understand there are a total of 125). Of the 122 schools, 98 responded to their survey with 95 providing detailed information. Of these 95, one indicated outright that they did not offer nutrition education, and 94 claimed to offer nutrition education. Of these 94 schools, 32 did not specify how their required nutrition was taught, 25 stated that nutrition was integrated into other courses, only 31 had stand-alone nutrition courses, and 6 had strictly optional nutrition education, which included library or independent study. This, then, indicated that 88 schools required some nutrition education.

Within these 88 schools, the courses in which nutrition was taught were designated as follows: Nutrition, 31; Biochemistry, 7; Physiology, 3; Integrated curriculum, 11; and Clinical practice, 4. In other words, only 31 had courses that included 'nutrition' in the title or description.

Even more revealing, however, is the reported number of hours of instruction in nutrition by each of the 88 schools. Twenty-five of the schools reported giving equal-to-or-less than 10 hours of instruction, 37 schools reported 11 – 20 hours, 17 gave 21 – 30 hours, 3 gave 31 – 40 hours, and *only 5 schools gave greater than 40 hours of nutrition education.*

At this point, I would like to say this: studying biochemistry or other biology courses in a medical curriculum is *not* the same as studying nutrition ... believe me, I know. For example, I took the 440-441 courses in biochemistry taught to the pre-med students at UH, and I also studied biochemistry as taught within our FSHN curriculum ... they are definitely *not* the same. And, even 40 hours of instruction is really nothing ... the beginning Nutrition 101 course alone provides over 50 hours of in-class instruction.

And so, where and how does a typical medical physician learn what they know about nutrition ?? I suggest that they receive their knowledge from the same sources that you do ... from the news of the day and from popular magazines, and from books found for sale at Barnes & Noble, Borders, or other popular book stores. Yes, it is true that they are better equipped to understand and interpret nutritional information, with their background in the biology sciences and chemistry, but it is only a matter of degree. While good textbooks in nutrition *are* available, they are not commonly so ... I have noticed that our typical bookstores do not stock good nutrition textbooks, especially for advanced nutrition, and I doubt that many physicians bother to take a trip to the university bookstore to actively search for good nutrition textbooks.

So, then, why are medical doctors thought to be experts on nutrition? A very good question.

Throughout my years of studying nutrition I have tried to understand this reluctance by the medical community to give nutrition its due priority status. I must admit that the answer is not fully clear to me, even now, but I do have some plausible insights. One clue comes from studying the history of medicine and nutrition.

The paradigm notion that disease comes from *outside* the body only ... the example of vitamin C

Walter Gratzer, in his fascinating review of the history of nutrition, in *Terrors of the Table,* (2005) explains that the roots of Western medicine, and nutrition, goes back to Hippocrates of Cos (fifth century BC), whose theory was based on the concept of the *four humors*. The four humors were thought to be bodily counterparts to the four elements: earth, air, fire, and water. The teachings of Hippocrates was later reinforced by Galen of Pergamum, who was revered as "The Prince of Physicians" (second century AD), whose doctrines were considered immutable for 15 centuries. Much can be said to explain this early view of medicine, which also included the first theory of nutrition, but one central tenet of the Galen paradigm was that disease and ill-health was caused by factors only from *outside* the body, not by malfunctions *within* ones physiology. When considering food (and its nutrients), Galen taught that poor health resulted from *excesses*, rather than deficiencies. For example, Gratzer reports that Galen bragged that his father had lived to 100 because he avoided eating fruit his entire life ... fruits were given the attributes of 'cold' and 'moist' and thought to cause diarrhea and fevers. It is amazing that this belief predominated for so many centuries ... probably contributing to much of the malnutrition and infant mortality during those times.

A historical example of how the doctrines of Hippocrates and Galen influenced nutrition is the case of vitamin C.

The deficiency disease condition caused by an insufficient intake of this essential nutrient is 'scurvy', which can be a truly hideous disease. In early Scotland it was called "blacklegs" because of bloody patches forming under the skin. It can cause rotting of the gums and loss of teeth ... and hair. A sufferer may characterize extreme lassitude, or constipation so persistent that surgery may be required, and the victim often emits an intolerable stench of putrefaction.

It is curious that only a very few species in the entire animal kingdom cannot produce their own vitamin C ... humans are one of this select group. Others in the group include the chimpanzee, the gorilla, the guinea pig, the fruit bat, and one species of birds. Each of these species are supplied with ample vitamin C in their environment, suggesting that somewhere in our humanoid ancestral history we too lived in an environment with ample vitamin C and thus lost our ability to produce our own. Humans lack the liver enzyme *gulonolactone-oxidase*, required to catalyze the last step in the metabolic pathway to produce vitamin C ... we possess the necessary metabolic apparatus and pathway except for the very final step. Your dog and cat, the horse, the cow, the elephant ... all can produce their own vitamin C ... but you cannot.

The saga of vitamin C is long and filled with historical intrigue, starting from when scurvy was first identified as a specific disease condition in the time of Hippocrates, and even before, until vitamin C was finally isolated as ascorbic acid ... white crystals derived from lemons, oranges, paprika, cabbage, and adrenal glands ... accomplished in the years 1928-31. Scurvy was often a major factor in the outcome of historical battles and epic voyages of exploration. It was an issue with the Crusaders of the Middle Ages. During Vasco da Gama's voyage to the Indies half of his crew died from scurvy. A four-year circumnavigation by Commodore Anson started with seven ships and 2,000 men and ended with only 600 men surviving ... 4 had been killed in battle, the rest were lost to scurvy. A report on the effect of the disease among British sailors during the 1700's concluded that 19 deaths in every 20 had been the result of scurvy (John Hammond, 1747). Scurvy has been reported as a major cause of death in countless historical scenarios: the Mormons making their way to Utah in the mid 1800's, the siege of Paris in 1870, the siege of Kut-el-Amara in 1916, during The Great War (WWI), among the prospectors during the California gold rush, and during episodes of war and famine even today.

We all know that vitamin C, or ascorbic acid, is readily available from fruits and vegetables. An intake of only 13 milligrams per day is enough to ward off the ravishes of scurvy. We know that scurvy is the result of a deficiency ... it is the inability of the body to function because it lacks a nutrient .. *not* because of a virus, or an infectious attack from outside the body, or an excess intake of some substance. Yet it was the insistence that scurvy was caused by such things that prevailed for many long centuries, retarding the discovery of its cure and blocking the knowledge of the foods that could be eaten to prevent it. Galen's theory of humors, supported by the high prevalence of scurvy among sailors, concluded that the condition was caused by 'bad air' ... the damp air of the oceans or within the dark bilges of ships ... or by the excess intake of salt. The notion that consuming citrus fruits could prevent scurvy was unthinkable ... according to Galen doctrine, citrus fruit was "the commonest cause of fevers and obstructions of the vital organs".

Gratzer writes that one of the earliest challenges to the prevailing wisdom of the era was a book entitled *The Chirurgeon's Mate*, written by John Woodall in 1617. He had advocated eating fruits as a cure for scurvy, but he and his theory was paid little heed. In 1747 a British naval surgeon named James Lind performed a clinical trial aboard the HMS Salisbury which illustrated the value of citrus fruits in preventing scurvy, but by the time of his death in 1794 he and the results of his study were all but forgotten. Captain Cook, and several physicians who followed his thinking, thought they had found a cure with 'sweetwort' in the 1770's.

But it wasn't until a Scottish naval doctor named Gilbert Blane advocated the intake of lime juice that scurvy finally became controllable. Blane had seen the results of scurvy while serving with the British navy in the Carribean during the war with France in the 1780's. During one 12 month period 60 seamen had died in battle in the Carribean, over 1600 from scurvy. Through his efforts scurvy became almost unknown among the British navy by the turn of the century. Laboratory work done by Harriette Chick and her team in 1918 and published in the medical journal, *The Lancet*, finally put all debate to rest, and it became accepted that something in limes prevented scurvy. It was the end of a 300 year struggle against an entrenched paradigm. Ten years later ascorbic acid was isolated and identified as the 'vitamin' in limes that could prevent scurvy.

What is truly amazing in all of this is how one paradigm, filled with such error and misinformation, could prevail over the minds of intelligent men (and women) so completely and for so long. It is a lesson to consider. And when one looks critically at the reluctance of today's medical community to 'look within' for explanations and cures of disease conditions … the intake of essential nutrients, for example … then one cannot help but conclude that today's medical science is suffering from a hangover of a previous, antiquidated paradigm.

How often have you heard a medical doctor explain that this or this condition, the actual cause unknown, is probably due to a virus or infection from an outside source? How often have you heard it explained that the condition is not because of a nutrient deficiency, but by *too much* of a nutrient, or an excessive intake of one substance or another? Could this thinking be a ghost from a paradigm long antiquidated?

This is a complete aside, and perhaps I should be scolded for stating it, but the Galen paradigm's preoccupation with outside factors and causes rather than looking within is paralleled by the prevailing religious doctrine of the same period. I am, of course, talking about Christianity. It is to be noted that while some religions such as Buddism and Hinduism teach that we seek knowledge, and salvation, from within, Christianity teaches that we seek knowledge and our salvation from outside sources.

The emphasis of seeking explanations and cures for disease conditions and ill-health from *outside*, and in turn choosing to subordinate or ignore influences that take place *within*, such as with metabolism of nutrients, then, is one characteristic of the prevailing medical science paradigm

Monopoly of information

Have you heard the question recently "Is this good for me?" or "Why is this bad for me?" or "Who do I believe". It seems that everyone would like answers to the many questions they face regarding the foods they eat and their personal health. Yet there seems to be a severe shortage of credible sources for information. The dietitians speak about supporting breast-feeding and trying to improve the school lunches, but know almost nothing about supplements and have only standard, ultra-conservative answers to your real concerns … and they are found only in the hospitals anyway. The nutritionists? Who are they ? and … Where are they ? The professors in the university, you say ? How do we talk to *them* ?

240

How about our public school teachers? One would think that it is here, in the public schools and within our primary education system, that we would be taught at least basic nutrition ... and have a chance to learn more advanced nutrition. And yes, our school teachers do try to incorporate matters of nutrition in such courses as home economics, public health, science courses, and physical education. But it is all surface stuff only, with the continuous repetition of "eat a variety of basic foods and maintain a balanced diet"!! At best it is treated as part of dietetics ... never as 'the science of nutrition'. Have you ever heard of a high school course actually entitiled 'nutrition' ? And what do school teachers really know about nutrition anyway ? Where and how did *they* learn what they do know ? Have you ever heard of nutrition being a required course for an education major ?

Oh yes, there are a lot of books on the bookstore shelves, but you have read many of them, and you are tired of being told that this or that author is "the foremost nutrition expert" in the world, or that this one single magic substance is the cure for everything. Where does one read to obtain truly subjective and accurate information ?

But it is much worse than just that. Not so long ago medical doctors wrote their prescriptions in Latin, so only he and his pharmacist knew what he was talking about ... you were purposely kept in the dark. Has this changed? As one close friend recently remarked ... now their writing is so awful that it's really just the same thing !! I wonder ? Then you discover that your medical doctor doesn't really seem to know very much about nutrition. No wonder ... he probably learned what he knows from the same source as you did ... the chances that he learned anything about nutrition from his pre-med days or while at medical school is remote, as I have explained in the previous section.

It gets even worse. Scientists and academics love to talk to themselves, or only to each other. There is almost nothing in their world to prompt them to talk to the public ... there is no obligation to do so, no established mechanism to do so ... and they don't know how to speak normal language anyway. In addition, the writings about their studies are circulated among their peers for review, and only among their peers. Debate and continued studies to support or refute an original study are kept within that circle of peers and within selected scientific journals. The journals, in return, have considerable selective power over what they choose to print, or which scientist to favor. It is a closed world, with prestige, jealousy, and power playing major roles. Much criticism has been directed to this distasteful situation, over many years. But little has been done to make improvements. Some critics have stated that the system allows for much biased and money-sponsored research to squeeze its way past the sensors. One example has been the enormous quantity of reported research and discussion within the journals supporting cow's milk as "nature's most perfect food", and the unabashed sponsorship by the dairy industry.

It is prudent, however, to recognize and pay tribute to the tremendous success that medical science has had in identifying and eradicating infectious disease and diseases that truly *do* have an outside source. This cannot be understated. The progress and success, especially in the past two centuries, has uplifted our human health, increased our longevity, and eradicated a long list of diseases.

At the same time, however, a re-appraisal of the conventional wisdom is long over-due ... it is time for a *paradigm shift.*

About the series: *The Nutrition Factor: A Bold New Perspective*

The series takes on the challenge of identifying the aged paradigm of the conventional wisdom in mainstream nutrition and medical science, and suggests that the time for a 'paradigm shift' is long overdue. In Part One the author presents his own research, which challenges the often heard paradigm statement that "we can obtain all our necessary nutrients by consuming a variety of basic foods and maintaining a balanced diet" and suggests that, contrary to the conventional wisdom, it is very difficult, if not impossible, to do so. Part Two then explores the important contributions by S.B. Eaton and Melvin Konner, and other scientists in the same field, showing that our ancestral diet and lifestyle was very different from that of today. The conclusions to these findings are that our physiologies are designed for a different food supply than the one currently provided, and that our food choices and the foods themselves need to be reassessed, re-examined, and improved. Part Three then reviews a large number of nutritional issues, re-examining them in the light of a *bold new perspective*, with numerous insights and analogies. These issues include the question of whether or not we should pursue a vegetarian diet; and new insights freshly explore our understanding of atherosclerosis, diabetes, cancer, and weight control.

242

How the discussion of milk fits in with the series

The discussion of milk consumption by humans fits the broader context and scope of the series as an example of a food that (a) was not a part of our ancestral nutritional environment, that (b) changed in its make-up over centuries of modification, and (c) because milk consumption is a vivid example of the tenacious adherence to a previous, questionable paradigm. The belief that milk and milk products is an important food choice for humans is so overwhelmingly entrenched in our Western culture that it occupies an almost sacred position in the conventional wisdom, or prevailing paradigm, of nutrition and modern medicine.

Conclusions and implications of the series

The conclusions of the series include (a) that there is a need to re-appraise our conventional wisdom regarding nutrition, (b) that medical science and the health care community need to give more attention and support to the study of nutrition, (c) that nutrition needs to be instated as a bona-fide and central part of medicine itself, and (d) that we need to critically examine the nature and characteristics of our modern food supply, its nutrient content, and its compatibility with our physiologies.

The implications are therefore far-reaching and enormous. New research needs to be encouraged … research that is objective, carried out with integrity and transparency, and with the researchers bravely accepting new challenges. We need to investigate the potential for improving the nutritional value of our foods and to adjust our food choices and eating habits in order to obtain better nutrition. The medical schools and pre-med curriculums need to be revised to include advanced study in nutrition, and nutrition needs to be a required subject of study.

A Rare Inspirational Insight

Before entering the UH undergraduate program in Food Science and Human Nutrition, I sought to 'test the waters' by auditing the one nutrition course that was required by the 4-year nursing students, as I mentioned above. Our instructor was a rare lady, indeed. She was from the faculty of the associated John Burns Medical School, yet she had an extensive background in nutrition. During the semester she often referred to her experience working in the field of international nutrition in several developing countries. On first day of class ... and I will never forget this ... she approached from the front, holding her hands high and using her fingers to simulate quotation marks, and made a wonderful statement. It was a statement that was an inspiration to me at the time, and continues to be an inspiration even now. It also sums up the 'bold new perspective' of this series in a single phrase.

Later, as student editor of the FSHN Newsletter, I ventured to ask her permission to quote her inspirational statement. She was horrified: "No, you cannot do that ... they would kick me out of the medical school !!"

What she had said, in that memorable moment, went like this: "Why nutrition ?" she asked, with her fingers high and fluttering, "Because we now know that, at least in the United States, *long term health care is nutrition* !!"

References for the Appendix

Eaton, B.S.; Shostak, M.; Konner, M.; *The Paleolithic Prescription,* Harper & Row Publishers, 1988

Gratzer, W.; *Terrors of the Table: The Curious History of Nutrition,* Oxford University Press, 2005

Harris, M.; *Good to Eat, Riddles of Food and Culture,* Waveland Press, Inc. 1985, revised 1998

Kuhn, T.S.; *The Copernican Revolution, Planetary Astronomy in the Development of Western Thought,* Harvard University Press, 1957, 1985

Kuhn, T.S; *The Structure of Scientific Revolutions,* University of Chicago Press, 1962, 1970, 1996

Torti, Frank M. Jr.; Adams, Kelly M. MPH, RD; Edwards, Lloyd J., PhD; Lindell, Karen C., MS, RD; Zeissel, Steven H., MD, PhD; *Survery of Nutrition Education in U.S. Medical Schools – An Instructor-Based Analysis*, Department of Nutrition, University of North Carolina at Chapel Hill, Medical Education Online, http://www.med-ed-online.org/res00023.htm).

INDEX

About the author

His friends teased him mercilessly … "Don't go to his house for lunch … his mother will feed you meatless hotdogs and carrot juice!" Then there was the time the high-school principle told him to stay home for a few days because of the over-whelming odor of garlic emanating from his torso … Brent had had a cold, and phoned his mom in her health food store at the Bonnie Doon Shopping Center to ask what to do for it. She told him to take some garlic … so he enthusiastically gobbled up a large quantity, placing the cloves between slices of whole wheat bread. He never did hear the end of that one!

A few years later Brent left his parent's home in Edmonton, resolved not to have anything more to do with "health foods" and all the other nonsense that his mother tried to stuff him with. But an ever-present infatuation with the subject of nutrition continued to dog him, and his interest peaked anew when he had his own babies to care for, and wanted to give them the best nutrition possible. Without really knowing it, Brent had embarked on a life-long search for objective and unbiased knowledge in nutrition.

Just before his mother died in 1986, she sat down with him and talked about nutrition. She was a very disappointed woman at that time. She had devoted most of her life to learning about nutrition, and trying to help people with her knowledge. But her success had been only limited … every single cancer sufferer she had worked with finally died of cancer, and her own health had always been a problem, starting with diabetes when she was just a young girl. But she over-flowed with tremendous faith, and tried to pass some of it on to her son. His mother suggested that he go back to university and apply his ample learning skills to the field of nutrition. She re-iterated what he already knew … that the field of nutrition, at least in Canada and the U.S., was starkly divided into two opposing camps. On one side was nutrition as formally studied in the universities and copyrighted by the medical doctors and professional dietitians and nutritionists. The other was the world of 'health foods' and supplements and alternative medicine. But Kathryn Bateman had a vision. She told Brent that there *was* a middle road … that yes, there was a lot of misinformation and nonsense … on both sides … but that a more correct nutritional perspective lay somewhere in-between, and she challenged her son to re-enter the ivory towers and seek that middle path.

249

So he did just that, but found himself struggling an up-hill battle. He learned very quickly that having grown up in a health food store was not something to brag about, and that it was best to keep his insights from that exposure a secret. But it eventually leaked out, and, combined with his outspokenness and questioning attitude, his academic ambitions suffered. First, he was refused continued study at the University of Hawaii in the master's program in nutrition, although he had earned top grades in the undergraduate program in the same department, and had already been in the master's program one full semester. It was apparent that it had a lot to do with his proposed thesis topic, which was to create a computer program to test the paradigm statement that "you can obtain all your required nutrients by eating a variety of basic foods and maintaining a balanced diet". This was viewed as an unsuitable topic for a student wishing to gain membership to the nutritionist's exclusive 'club'. A number of other criticisms had surfaced. Brent had been the student editor of the FSHN Newsletter, and had been outspoken. In his editorials he had dared to question some of the basic tenets of the conventional wisdom in nutrition and modern medicine. In class Brent had once objected to milk as "the perfect food" and had mentioned a study, just published, that something in cow's milk caused an auto-immune reaction which prompted T-cells to attack the beta cells in the pancreas. His professor had told him that, quite frankly, he was "nuts". For one of his presentations he chose the study by Eaton and Konner of the Paleolithic diet. Finally, the newly appointed advisor to the post-graduate acceptance committee was stanchly against supplements of any kind, and Brent had spoken up in that professor's undergraduate class in favor of supplements. Although Brent had received an "A" in that class, the professor made it clear that his pro-supplement attitude was "unacceptable". He was then told by this gentleman's close colleague that he "should choose another field of study".

Maybe being forced to leave the University of Hawaii program was a blessing, because Brent then discovered the Institute of Nutrition at Mahidol University in Thailand ... an institute with a truly international perspective and curriculum, and a prestigious reputation. Ironically, he made this discovery via the same professor that told him he should seek another field of study. Brent was more careful this round, however, and chose a different thesis topic ... and was very hush-hush about his experiences at the University of Hawaii, and his more distant health food past. The director of the institute, and Brent's mentor, Dr. Kraisid Tontisirin, had known that Brent also possessed a B.A. in Economics, and suggested that his thesis combine economics and nutrition. Brent followed his advice, entitling the thesis "Nutriton Intervention: A Potential Factor For Economic Growth and Development". It was a great topic. But Dr. Kraisid left INMU shortly after Brent started on his thesis, becoming the director of the Food Policy and Nutrition Division of the FAO, The United Nations, stationed in Rome. Brent was required to find another advisor, and was passed from professor to professor; ending up with ... wouldn't you believe it ... a professor who was a good friend of his antagonist at the University of Hawaii ... they had studied and received their PhD's together at Cornell. Once again he was under fire.

One of Brent's good friends, also from UH, coached him to be steadfast and to persevere. He re-wrote that 200 page thesis, end-to-end, fifteen separate times ... and it took three years of relentless effort. On the final day, after having successfully defended the thesis and meeting with his advisor for one last time ... she asked Brent what he wanted to do ... what were his plans. Brent told her he wanted to continue to study nutrition, and to write about nutrition. Her face darkened. She said "Brent, I know you 'come from the other side'. I hope you don't write anything to hurt us." To this day Brent wonders at that statement, and all its implications, and is amazed that it was made by a PhD in nutrition.

During the frequent empty spaces of time waiting for his Mahidol thesis advisor to review his latest version and tell him to re-write it all once again, Brent travelled throughout Thailand, exploring every corner. He fell in love with the picturesque border town of Sangkhlaburi, located at the northern end of the Khao Laem lake in Kanchanaburi Province. He was astonished to see that there were no boats on the lake, so decided to make Sangkhlaburi his new home and open a small shop building North American style wooden canoes and kayaks. Brent encourages the reader to visit his website to learn more about his boat shop at www.sanghaleicanoeandkayak.com. Besides taking care of his boat shop and writing, Brent has opened a sewing factory to support his once-upon-a-time secretary's dress-making business in Honolulu, is converting a Phraya River rice barge to a beautiful lake launch, and is opening a restaurant.

But even will all that, Brent has also found new directions to explore in nutrition and human health. One dream is to continue studying in a university setting ... the University of Chulalongkhan offers a PhD curriculum for international students in Public Health, with a specialty in nutrition. Brent is also working with a group of ethnic Mon and Karen friends to learn about the vast diversity of plants used by the indigenous peoples of Thailand and Myanmar, and is putting together a book in an

251

effort to preserve their vulnerable knowledge. He is also deeply interested in Thai Traditional Medicine and Thai Traditional Massage. Who knows … he may one day open a health/nutrition spa in his hide-away home alongside the beautiful Khao Laem lake.

Although this is Brent's first book on the topic of nutrition, he hopes to continue writing on this favorite topic, and has outlined a series which he has entitled *The Nutrition Factor: A Bold New Perspective.*

But this is not his very first book, however. He self-published *The Last Voyage of the New Guinea Trader* in 2003 … a mischievous true-life account of one of his adventures while travelling the globe in his younger years. Brent also acted as writer, editor, and agent for his dear friend, Rex Gunn, who passed away in 1999. Rex had been a G.I. and war correspondent during the WWII 'war in the Pacific' and had left behind severl manuscripts, which Brent edited, re-wrote, and published. One was *Suddenly .. On A Sunday Morning*, an account of the bombing of Pearl Harbor; another was *They Called Her Tokyo Rose*, the telling of the tragic story of Iva Toguri, wrongly convicted as a the traitor, Tokyo Rose.

www.ingramcontent.com/pod-product-compliance
Lightning Source LLC
Chambersburg PA
CBHW060840280326

41934CB00007B/855